Your Survival Guide to Cosmetic Surgery

ANTHONY N. LABRUNA, M.D., F.A.C.S.,
& JACLYN MUCARIA, M.P.A.

YOUR SURVIVAL GUIDE TO COSMETIC SURGERY

2007

Your Survival Guide to Cosmetic Surgery

TABLE OF CONTENTS

INTRODUCTION

I s anyone happy with the way they look anymore? Anyone can see that cosmetic surgery is a booming business with increasing popularity. In any given week, you can tune into reality television shows or read articles and books on this topic. Once a taboo subject, it has now become acceptable to undergo, and even talk freely about cosmetic surgery. Recently, many celebrities have gone public by revealing their new faces or bodies and speaking explicitly about their surgical procedure. Like it or not, plastic surgery (also referred to as cosmetic surgery) is more than a passing fad, and people cannot seem to get enough information on this topic.

According to data published by the American Society for Aesthetic Plastic Surgery, there were 11.5 million surgical and non-surgical cosmetic procedures performed in this country in 2006, a 44% increase from only two years year before! This whopping increase indicates that more and more people are turning to cosmetic and reconstructive procedures to make a positive impact on their lives.

The American Society for Aesthetic Plastic Surgery data reported that the top five cosmetic surgical procedures in 2006 were liposuction (403,684), breast augmentation (383,886), eye procedures (209,999), abdominoplasty (tummy tuck) (172,457) and breast reduction (145,822). Surgical procedures accounted for nearly 17% of the total procedures.

The top five non-surgical procedures in 2006 were Botox® (3,181,592), hyaluronic acid (1,593,554) laser hair removal (1,475,296), microdermabrasion (993,071), and laser skin resurfacing (576,509). Women had nearly 10,500,000 cosmetic procedures in 2006 accounting for 92 % of the total. The 35-50 age group accounted for 47 % of all cosmetic surgery procedures, ages 51-64 accounted for 25 %, ages 19—34 accounted for 22 %, and those over 65 had 5 % of the procedures.

Since 1997, surgical procedures increased 123 %, while non-surgical procedures have increased 749 %.

As these statistics illustrate, millions of people are making decisions each year to have cosmetic surgery. The selection of a surgeon, planning for the procedure and recovery period, and setting realistic expectations can be a daunting task for many people. This book was created to help you navigate your way through through the system and make the right decisions.

Why Is This Book Different?

Your Survival Guide to Cosmetic Surgery was written to assist the millions of people who are contemplating cosmetic surgery and could benefit from practical information from experts in the field. You will get direct and honest answers to all of your questions (including those that you were afraid to ask, or haven't even thought of yet). This book will walk you through the various phases of the process: making your decision to have surgery, various surgical and non-surgical options, selecting your surgeon, getting the most out of your consultation, preparing for surgery, and planning for your recovery. All photographs, questions, and quotes in this book are from actual patients; all responses and opinions are those of an expert doubly board certified plastic surgeon.

As the title suggests, this book will be a tell-all guide; an invaluable resource with tips, secrets, success stories, and expert knowledge. The objective of the guide is not to be a quick read and find its rightful place on your bookshelf. You will appreciate this guide most if you carry it with you through every phase of your procedure, and for many weeks and months afterward.

Cosmetic surgery is extremely popular and can open up many doors by giving people a new sense of confidence and well-being. Unfortunately, if done for the wrong reasons, this surgery can lead to disappointment. In your consultation, the surgeon will review with you in detail what physical attributes you are looking to change and what options are available. It is extremely important for a surgeon to employ a holistic approach to a patient's evaluation. A holistic approach will involve an extensive discussion on all facets of the patient's life, such as relationships, career goals, responsibilities, support systems at home, timeframe, and a long-term aesthetic plan. The chapter "What To Expect At Your Consultation" will go into more detail on the holistic approach.

In some chapters, you will notice questions with their respective responses. The questions have been collected from patients over the course of several years. You will quickly notice that all responses are brief and to the point, some may even be somewhat provocative—but all are truthful and will be of great value to you in your journey. You should also note that in the book, we regard the terms "cosmetic surgery" and "plastic surgery" as synonymous. There is no difference between the two terms.

Hopefully, this book will answer the myriad questions that you may have while thinking about a cosmetic improvement.

CHAPTER 1
Why Do You Think You Need Cosmetic Surgery?

Everyday, millions of people look in the mirror and are not satisfied with what they see. Many of them turn to cosmetic procedures to improve their appearance. As a result, there were more than eight million cosmetic procedures performed in the U.S. last year. There are numerous reasons why people desire cosmetic improvements. Some people do it for the right reasons and others for the wrong reasons. Physicians should ask patients probing questions and in return, patients should provide open and honest responses. This dialogue and rapport are an essential component of a successful patient-physician relationship.

When you meet your prospective surgeon, he or she will ask you what you intend to change and why are you looking for this change. This conversation is very important in determining what may occur in the future. If your surgeon does not spend enough time with you or rushes you through the process, it may be time to select another physician. Some patients are convinced that surgery will solve all of their problems, or that beauty will make them happier. It has been demonstrated that patients having procedures for the wrong reasons are likely to be disappointed later. It is critical that both parties (patient and surgeon) understand and agree on what the surgery will accomplish.

In your consultation, you will use a number of criteria (which we will provide later) to "size up" the surgeon. You may not be aware, however, that in this discussion, the surgeon is also evaluating you. Some patients are ideal candidates for surgery and others are not. As you will learn, not every patient is an ideal candidate for surgery, and some may even be discouraged by their physician.

Most patients seeking cosmetic procedures have done research, have a well thought out plan, and are great candidates for surgery. There is, however, a subset of patients for whom surgery is not the answer. An experienced plastic surgeon will not accept a patient who has unrealistic expectations or for whom the risk is higher than the reward.

Over the years and seeing thousands of prospective patients, we have found that they fall into several common categories.

*The **Realist:*** These people are well-balanced and happy with life. They are comfortable with their appearance, but are dissatisfied with a specific physical feature. It is their perception that this imperfection compromises their self-image and confidence. They have considered options, including surgery, and have done their research. They have digested heaps of information and have the financial resources to proceed. They have reasonable expectations about what can be done to improve their appearance and are not looking for a miracle cure. *The **Realist** is an ideal candidate for cosmetic surgery.*

*The **Business Person:*** These people want to improve something in order to gain something else. Surgery is a means to an end—examples could be a new job, more corporate earning power, a leading role in a play. Typical ***Business People*** may be dancers, waitresses, strippers, or any other occupation where good looks are a key success factor. These people possess high levels of self—esteem, but feel that some physical attribute is standing between them and their desired goal. In these cases, cosmetic surgery can do two things: it can improve them physically, but can also result in building confidence which could lead to the desired outcome. The Baby Boomer would be placed in the ***Business Person*** group. Typical Baby Boomers have achieved success, but view surgery as a tool to extend or enhance their career goals. Baby Boomers, typically in their forties and fifties, feel much younger but see their face or body showing signs of aging. More than likely, the ***Business Person*** has the financial resources and the time to move ahead with their decision for surgery. The ***Business Person*** *is an excellent candidate for surgery as long as he/she is realistic with manageable expectations.*

*The **Accommodator:*** These people desire surgery solely to please someone else. Typically, they lack self—esteem or have relationship problems and are convinced that cosmetic surgery is a panacea. For example, the *Accommodator* may want a face lift, or larger breasts only because it would make their spouse happier. When asked, these patients may not be unhappy with their appearance, but have a greater need to impress their significant other. The decision to have surgery, in these cases, is one made under pressure, or stemming from a strong desire to please. The *Accommodator* often learns too late that surgery was not the answer. As a result, they may experience stress or depression after the procedure, irrespective of the result. Every surgical procedure, however minor, has risks and should never be taken lightly. One should never undergo cosmetic surgery to gain acceptance from someone else. The desire for improvement should come from within. *Accommodators may not the best candidates for surgery if they are not in full agreement that an improvement is necessary. They must want the change to please themselves, not someone else.*

The Perfectionist: These patients are never satisfied with their result. They either have unrealistic expectations or seek a level of unachievable perfection. A typical *Perfectionist* carries a gorgeous celebrity's photograph to the surgeon's office. Although most of us would love to have Angelina Jolie's lips, Tom Cruise's eyes, or Brad Pitt's smile, the *Perfectionist* will not be satisfied until they believe they have it. They may have the same procedure performed over and over, sometimes by several different surgeons trying to achieve the result that they desire. The *Perfectionist* is a challenge for the surgeon because the surgery will likely be followed by disappointment. These patients sometimes threaten to sue the surgeon because the outcome did not match their expectation. It is the responsibility of the surgeon to discuss openly and honestly what can and cannot be done for a patient. It is important to remember that even the most experienced surgeon cannot produce a miracle. *Unless these Perfectionists can lower their expectations, they will never be ideal candidates for surgery.*

The Pushy Parent: This is a common scenario where the parent decides unilaterally that a child requires surgery. Similar to the *Perfectionist*, the *Pushy Parent* wants a perfect child. A problem arises, however, when the child does not want surgery, or does not understand the implications. Often, **Pushy Parents** seek surgery in order to satisfy their own needs, rather than those of their child. It is critical to note that not all parents seeking surgery for their child fall under the category of **Pushy Parent**. There are situations where a parent correctly identifies a problem, and appropriately seeks intervention. One example is a child with a deformity or other physical imperfection. This child may lose self-confidence, become depressed, or be frequently ridiculed in school. The child and parent do their research, perhaps consult a psychologist, then decide together that surgery is the best solution. This is a very different scenario than the **Pushy Parent**, who insists on a nose job for a young child simply because the parent does not like their child's nose. We also hear of mothers who request breast implants for their daughters even when they are in their teens. It is important for the surgeon to gain the trust and confidence of the child to fully understand the situation before any decision is made. An insightful surgeon will elicit the child's opinion about their desire for surgery. *The child of the **Pushy Parent** may not be an ideal candidate for surgery unless he/she agrees with the decision and can understand all of the implications.*

The Professional Patient: Everyone can name someone who appears to have had one cosmetic procedure too many! These patients are hooked and never satisfied with a slight improvement; they want a total body overhaul! Typically, they have low self—esteem and are unhappy with themselves. They can never have enough surgery; the more they have, the more they crave. The *Professional Patient* recovers from one procedure, only to seek another one. The typical *Professional Patient* will change their eyes and nose, then, several months later, move on to the face, breasts, and tummy. The ethical plastic surgeon will understand what is driving this patient and will not perform unnecessary surgery. Some of these patients would benefit more from counseling rather than more surgery. *The **Professional Patient** is not always a bad candidate for surgery, but must be carefully managed by their surgeon to avoid overindulgence.*

One of the most important factors in making your decision is to have an honest discussion with your surgeon and yourself. Both you and your surgeon should agree on what will be done, how it will be done, and what results to expect. This agreement on both sides will lessen the likelihood of any disappointment later in the process.

"How will I know if I am making the right decision?"

Trust your gut instinct. If you are well informed, fully understand the risks and benefits, and what improvements are possible; you have likely made the right decision. If you fall into one of the categories of patients who are not ideal candidates, you may want to revisit the reasons for wanting cosmetic surgery. The decision you make must be the right one for you!

CHAPTER 2
Now You're Ready!

We have no doubt that you have seen face lifts that have gone too far, or a nose job just doesn't look right. It is clear that patients can end up with awful results because they chose the wrong surgeon. Although there is no way to guarantee great results, the match between the patient and surgeon is a key factor to success. (You will hear this message in many parts of this book.) This chapter will equip you with tips and secrets to finding the best surgeon for you.

Take Your Time

The more information you collect ahead of time, the more prepared you will be to make your decision. Since cosmetic surgery is elective, you have the luxury of time to do your homework. It is your responsibility to take time with your decision. Do not be lured in by full-page advertisements or low fees. Selecting a cosmetic surgeon is the beginning of an expensive and long-term commitment. Do not look for shortcuts. Interestingly enough, the same person who will do exhaustive research and multiple test drives before buying a car will choose a surgeon from the yellow pages or a subway advertisement. Unfortunately, once some people decide that they want surgery, they want it scheduled as soon as possible. This is an unrealistic and irresponsible approach that can lead to disaster. There is a wealth of valuable information out there. It takes significant time and energy to collect, organize and understand this information. If you cannot do this alone, enlist a friend to help organize and narrow the field.

Deciphering Credentials and Certifications

Most people are not well-versed in physician credentialing and can easily be mislead. This is an important section for you to understand as you muddle thorough the morass of initials, societies, boards, and degrees. While we want to give you enough information to help you in your search, we do not want to overwhelm you with jargon. After reading this section, you will quickly be able to evaluate your surgeon and focus on the "**must have**" credentials rather than the window dressing.

Board Certification

As you probably have discerned, the specialty of cosmetic surgery is a lucrative business. Some doctors are attracted to the field for the wrong reasons, or may not be qualified enough to call themselves cosmetic surgeons. Patients often look for the phrase "board certified" after a physician's name as some assurance of quality. Many do not know that board certification may be in a specialty that is far removed from cosmetic surgery. For example, a board certified obstetrician with years of experience in delivering babies decides to add tummy tucks and liposuction to his practice. A patient may not question this decision, since it still involves the abdomen and pelvis area. One must question, however, if certification in Obstetrics and Gynecology ensures that this physician is qualified to perform cosmetic procedures? The answer is a resounding NO. Even if this physician expertly delivered your baby and you trust him or her with your care, you should not assume that he or she is the best qualified when you are seeking cosmetic surgery.

The most important board certification that you should look for is from the American Board of Plastic Surgery (ABPS). The American Board of Plastic Surgery is one of the 24 specialty boards under the purview of the American Board of Medical Specialties (ABMS). The ABMS establishes the minimum standards for physician training, education, and experience. Physicians who possess the ABPS certification have been deemed qualified to perform reconstructive and cosmetic surgery. This certification is a "**must have**" when looking for your surgeon.

Plastic surgeons that are certified by the ABPS must complete a rigorous list of requirements:
- Graduate of an accredited medical school
- Completed at least three years of surgical residency training
- Completed an additional two to three years of residency training in plastic

- Meets moral and ethical standards set forth by the ABPS
- After two years of practice, MD must pass comprehensive written and oral examinations

You can call the American Board of Medical Specialties at 800-776-2378 to verify a physician's credentials. If the ABMS cannot confirm the board certification for your surgeon, you should probably keep looking!

On occasion, you will come across a physician who is "doubly board certified." This is a prestigious credential as it illustrates someone who has met all the requirements for two different accrediting boards. If a surgeon is board certified in plastic surgery and also certified in another field, that is usually a winning combination! This is not a "**must have**," but it is an impressive credential if you run across someone who has it.

There are other board certifications that are not designated by the American Board of Medical Specialties but can sound quite impressive. The requirements for entrance into these boards may not be as rigorous as the ABMS boards. These self-designated boards set their own standards for membership and there is great variation among them. Don't be fooled into thinking a doctor is an expert if he or she is a member of these boards. Participation in these boards must be in addition to the American Board of Plastic Surgery, not instead of it.

Societies
There are other professional associations to which physicians belong and often use as part of their credentials. These are generally a good thing to look for when researching credentials. Many of the societies promote high standards and education through conferences, newsletters, and journals. The two most common societies for plastic surgery are the American Society of Plastic and Reconstructive Surgery and the American Society for Aesthetic Plastic Surgery. Only physicians who are board certified in plastic surgery are permitted to join these societies.

The American Society of Plastic Surgeons is a non-profit organization that supports their members toward their goal of providing the best patient care, education and research. The ASPS offers the most comprehensive, reliable data on plastic surgery procedures. Representing 94% of all the board-certified plastic surgeons in the U.S., the ASPS is a valuable source of information on new techniques, trends, and statistical data.

Hospital Affiliations

You may think that hospitals are for the sick, and you are not sick. Even if your surgeon performs most of the surgery in a private office, you should research his or her hospital privileges. In order for a physician to operate in a hospital or admit you if you have a complication, he or she must have admitting privileges. Physicians applying for hospital privileges must meet certain requirements established by their department. Hospitals and clinical departments have strict policies and procedures to ensure the clinical, academic, ethical, and moral standards for the physicians on their staff. These policies help to weed out the physician who does not have the required training or experience. It is rare to find a surgeon who does not have any hospital affiliations at all. If you do run across such a surgeon, be very wary since this is not a good sign.

Once you have determined the hospital affiliation, find out if the institution is reputable. Would you have a choice of hospitals, or only one? Is this a hospital that you or a family member has been treated in the past? All of these are important questions to ask in your process. Although a hospital affiliation does not guarantee excellence, it is a "**must have**," in our opinion, when choosing a surgeon.

Asking Around

If you do not intend to keep your surgery a secret, one of the best ways to find a great doctor is by personal recommendation. If a good friend conducted their own research and was thrilled with the results, that's a good starting point. If someone you know was pleased, that increases the likelihood that you will be pleased as well. Do not misunderstand this point. This is not a shortcut. A referral does not mean that you should skimp on doing your own research; it may just help you later as you narrow down your list.

Other excellent referral sources are the physicians, nurses, or other medical professionals who have witnessed the surgeon's work. Everyday, there are countless procedures done in hospitals and free-standing centers.

If you are lucky enough to know staff who work in these facilities, you can often get the inside scoop on surgeons. Some questions you should ask are:

- Is this surgeon skilled in the operating room?
- Does he or she perform the surgery themselves?
- How does he or she interact with patients?
- How is the response in emergencies?
- Are the patients satisfied with their results?
- Is this procedure something he or she performs often?
- Is this surgeon known to be available and approachable?
- Do other patients refer to this surgeon?

This is invaluable information if you are fortunate enough to get it. Many cosmetic surgery patients prefer privacy and choose not to publicize their search for a surgeon. Although this becomes a bit more challenging, it is not impossible to find the right doctor for you.

What About Advertisements, Internet or Telephone Directories?
There are two words that come to mind when someone obtains a physician's name from the phone directory or internet: **Be Careful.** While all of these venues are viable options to get names of surgeons, you should use them with extreme caution. As scary as it sounds, anyone with a medical degree and license can perform surgery. People can mislead the public by advertising themselves as experts when they lack the training or experience. Full page ads in the yellow pages will catch your eye and glossy magazine ads are very alluring. Some physicians even hire public relations firms to get their name out to the public. We do not recommend choosing your physician by the size or appearance of an advertisement. We are in no way implying that all physicians who advertise should be ruled out. What we are saying is that information from ads should be used in concert with all of the other information you have gathered to form your decision.

The internet is a Godsend if used correctly. It is a common practice for physicians to create their own web sites describing their experience, education, and credentials. These sites are usually informative and although they can be very helpful, we warn, "buyer beware." There are no checks and balances in the web world which guarantee truthful information. More reliable sources are the professional boards, societies, medical schools, and hospital web sites. These sites are more quality controlled and allow easy access to names of physicians grouped by specialty, location, credentials insurance, or gender.

The Final Few

You've asked around, conducted some research, and collected a list of names. After evaluating their credentials, you should be able to narrow the list and schedule your consultation appointments. In the next chapter, we will tell you what to expect at your first visit. Perhaps you've reduced the list to one clear favorite, but more than likely, you have two or three possibilities. To keep the process manageable, we do not recommend extensive window shopping. If you have done your homework correctly, each surgeon on your short list will have acceptable credentials. At this stage, the face to face meeting will be an important determining factor.

"I want my eyes done and asked my ophthalmologist for a referral. He says that he can do it himself, and I don't need a plastic surgeon. What should I do?"

Would you allow this ophthalmologist to deliver your baby? No! You need to conduct a bit of research before making a decision. If this ophthalmologist has the appropriate credentials and training, and you feel comfortable with him or her, go ahead. Perhaps you have stumbled upon a rare physician who is doubly board certified and is fully qualified to perform your surgery. Our advice, however, is to be careful; do not take a shortcut. Just because this doctor is a great ophthalmologist does not mean that he or she is qualified to do a blepharoplasty. Although it is not the norm, there are physicians who call themselves qualified because they completed a weekend course in cosmetics. Even though you are already a patient, do not (**under any circumstances**) allow the physician to perform surgery outside of their field until you do your homework. Only if the physician has fulfilled all of the training requirements and is board certified in plastic surgery should you proceed.

CHAPTER 3
What To Expect At Your Consultation

Now that you have narrowed your list down to a manageable few, it is time to meet the physicians face to face. This chapter will give you vital questions to ask and hints about how to finalize your decision to have surgery, and by whom.

What Is a Consultation and Why Is it So Important?

The purpose of the consultation is to meet face to face with the surgeon to see if you feel comfortable with him or her. This meeting is critical because, after your discussion, you will likely make a decision whether to proceed, ponder your decision a while longer, or keep looking. You may not realize it, but the physician is also evaluating you as a potential surgical candidate: Are your expectations realistic? Are there co-existing conditions that will make surgery difficult? Will you be compliant with post-operative instructions? Similar to a job interview, this thirty minute meeting may determine the future. The recipe for compatibility is part communication, part mutual respect and part rapport. Good compatibility and mutual trust will facilitate the entire surgical and recovery process.

In order to for your consultation to be successful, you must communicate effectively in a bi-directional manner with your physician. One person should not dominate the conversation or evade any topics. By this point, you have already conducted your research and have a list of questions. Patients who have done their homework and understand what is being told to them are the best candidates for surgery. Some patients get so star-struck by a wall full of diplomas, a luxurious office, or suave demeanor, that they forget their list of questions. Your physician should appear confident, honest, and knowledgeable without being arrogant or condescending. Any surgeon who guarantees results is not being honest with you. In medicine and surgery, there are likely outcomes and probabilities of success, but, unfortunately, there are no guarantees.

Evaluating Staff and Facilities

The physician can be viewed as the captain of the ship and controls all aspects of the voyage. The way that the office operates is a clear reflection of the surgeon and his expectations. You can begin your evaluation of the physician by the first phone contact with the office. How do they answer the phones? How were you welcomed at your appointment? Did the office appear to be organized? Did you wait excessively for your appointment? Were you greeted warmly? Was the environment clean and safe?

The office should be staffed with courteous, knowledgeable employees and should run smoothly and efficiently. The environment does not have to be luxurious, or in the most exclusive part of town. We would much prefer an office environment that is warm and inviting with knowledgeable staff to one that is luxurious and filled with antiques. You should be seen at or close to your scheduled appointment time. Since medical emergencies do occur, the staff should advise you if the physician is delayed. Extensive delays should be communicated with an option to reschedule the appointment if necessary. Most patients will not mind waiting if they are kept informed of the physician's estimated time of arrival.

Different surgeons staff their office to suit their practice. You may be seen by a receptionist, biller, nurse, medical assistant, and the surgeon. Each person should be professional, courteous, and knowledgeable as they interact with you, the patient. Your privacy and confidentiality **must** be provided at every point in the visit.

The Holistic Evaluation

As mentioned in the introduction, it is highly important for your surgeon to explore the various facets of your life. Cosmetic surgery is an art which, if used correctly, will yield a great aesthetic improvement. The holistic evaluation, if performed correctly, will include an exploration of the following topics:

- Timeframe: When is the optimal time for surgery? Can you schedule recovery time? When can you take off from work? Does season play a role?
- Support System: Who will be at home to take care of you for three days? Do you need a professional nurse? Even loving family members may not be the most helpful after surgery
- Geographic location: Where do you plan to stay after surgery? How far do you have to travel? How long do you need to stay locally for follow-up appointments?
- Career: Patients in certain careers, like stock brokers only want to know how fast they can get back on the phone, while other jobs have a large degree of face to face contact. Your career may have a direct impact on the technique used, as well as the desired outcome.
- Personal relationships: The decision to have surgery sometimes results from changes in one's relationship, desire for a new relationship, or pressure from a significant other. Sometimes, surgery is requested only to impress someone else. These relationships that impact a patient's desire for surgery should be explored and discussed.
- Long-term cosmetic goal: Many patients who embark on this cosmetic journey may choose to have several procedures over the course of many years. The timing and coordination of these procedures is important for the surgeon to plan.
- General physical and emotional health: The surgeon will likely ask you general questions about your life. He is trying to ascertain whether or not you are a good candidate for surgery. How will you react if the outcome is not what you expected? Or if you suffer a complication? Will you follow instructions and be compliant in your recovery process? All of these will be important factors in the decision making process.

The Treatment Plan

On your fist visit, the physician will typically ask "What can I do for you?" or "What brings you here today?" This is your opportunity to definitively describe what bothers you and what you hope to achieve with surgery. The surgeon will then do an examination and evaluation.

Surgical and possible non-surgical options will be discussed. It is common for the surgeon to recommend additional procedures related to the area of focus. For example, if a patient wants their nose reduced, the surgeon may suggest adding a chin implant to create a balanced look on the face. Recommending this related procedure is appropriate and provides the patient with options. On the other hand, you need to be skeptical if a physician recommends totally unrelated procedures or appears to be drumming up business. Some physicians may also suggest that the procedures can be discounted or save time if performed simultaneously. This is bad advice; remember that no surgery is without risk. If your surgeon recommends additional work, it is your responsibility to fully discuss and understand the reasons for doing so. Some patients are vulnerable and will concede to whatever the surgeon suggests, even if it is not appropriate. Hopefully, this scenario does not happen too often, but we wanted you to be aware that it does exist and to be careful.

When discussing the treatment plan, the physician will review the following:

- Recommended surgery to correct the problem
- Possible non-invasive options
- Surgical technique
- Location of incisions
- Duration of the procedure
- Post operative recovery period
- Level of pain to be expected
- Risks associated with the specific procedure
- Possible complications
- What to expect after surgery
- How long before you can return to work
- How long before you will see the full benefit of the surgery
- How long the improvement will last

All of this information can be overwhelming, so we suggest that you take notes. Many patients bring someone with them who can help with the details of the conversation. It is important for you to go home and distill all of the information in order to make an informed decision. Most surgeons will encourage you to take time with your decision, even if you verbalize your intent to proceed. Beware of the physician who pressures you to schedule your surgery immediately, before you've had a chance to think it over.

Medical History and Risk Assessment

When evaluating you as a potential surgical candidate, the surgeon will ask many questions regarding your medical history. This is not the time to withhold any information. The surgeon will want to discuss all past significant medical and surgical history, allergies, medications, and smoking and drinking habits. It is also important to disclose any supplements or herbs that you are taking, as they may interfere with the surgery or post op recovery. We will talk about herbs and supplements in a later chapter. If you take several medications, it may be helpful to bring a list with you to give to the physician so it can be part of your medical record. A detailed history is vital because the treatment plan, potential risks, type of anesthesia, even the location of the surgery will be based upon this personal information.

Photographs

Photographs are an essential part of the surgical consultation. These photographs will become an official part of your medical record. " Before" and "After" photos have become standard practice and are used to assess the changes that result from the cosmetic surgery. It is common for the surgeon and patient to refer to these photos throughout their pre-surgical and post-operative process. Many patients forget what they looked like before the surgery, and may question the degree of improvement. They may not see enough of a change and think the surgery was not successful. Most often, when the surgeon shows them their "Before" photos, they are usually pleasantly surprised with their result.

On occasion, patients ask to see "Before" and "After" photographs of other patients. Disclosing another patient's information or photographs is a violation of confidentiality unless the patient consents. Even if the surgeon obtains consent, it is our opinion that viewing other patients' successes is overrated. Another patient's result may be helpful, but it should not be represented as a guarantee of your outcome.

Computer Imaging

Patients frequently request computer imaging as a predictor of their outcome. Many surgeons have this technology in their office, and the honest surgeon will use it with caution. Imaging can illustrate the surgical possibilities, but may not be reflective of the actual result. Some physicians and patients are impressed with this technology. Using it cautiously can be fun and educational since different options and procedures can be viewed. For example, you can see what your nose may look like without the bump or what your brows will look like after the lift. Similar to the discussion on other patients' photos, these computer images are not a guarantee of your result. Patients frequently ask for this tool, and may be impressed if the physician has it, but it should not be overrated.

Location and Anesthesia

At your consultation, the surgeon will review the different types of anesthesia appropriate for your procedure. He or she may also offer various locations in which to have the surgery. Procedures can be performed in a private office, ambulatory surgery center, or a hospital. Many surgeons routinely operate in all three locations depending on the procedure and the patient's desire. There are advantages and disadvantages associated with each location. In the next chapter, we will provide the pros and cons of each type of facility and how to decide which one is appropriate for you. There are also several types of anesthesia that the surgeon may elect to use. This is an extremely important topic that we will review later on in the "Survival Guide."

Understanding the Cost of Surgery

Cosmetic surgery is not inexpensive and is an elective procedure. A fundamental question you need to ask yourself is, "Can I afford to have this surgery?" Before getting too far down the road, you must make this decision. A full understanding of fee arrangement is an important factor in evaluating whether or not to proceed.

Fees should be discussed in detail at your consultation either by the physician or billing representative. There are several fees that comprise the total cost of the surgery. This fact is not always made clear to the patient and may lead to confusion later. When given a quote for your procedure, you must be fully aware of what is and is not included. If a physician quotes his or her fee alone, you are not getting the full picture. Patients who have done their research will likely ask for a detailed quote that includes the total cost of the surgery.

The overall cost of surgery includes a surgeon's fee, anesthesiologist's fee, and an operating room (facility) fee. Some cases, like breast augmentations or chin enhancements, may also have a separate implant fee. Since these fees can range from several hundred to several thousand dollars each, the total cost of surgery is not insignificant. Of course, fees vary by surgeon, facility, and geography. Cities like New York and Beverly Hills command higher fees than the rest of the country. We will list specific fees in the next chapter.

Cosmetic surgery is considered a luxury item and is usually not covered by insurance. In certain cases, when the surgery corrects a malformation or deformity, the physician may request payment from the insurance company. For example, a breast reduction to reduce back pain may be covered by insurance. Reconstructive surgery or skin grafts following removal of a cancerous tumor may also be covered by insurance. These instances, however, are exceptions to the rule. For the majority of cosmetic surgery, the full financial burden is borne by the patient. On occasion, patients ask their surgeon to falsely justify their cosmetic procedure to the insurance company. Without realizing it, these patients are asking their surgeon to commit fraud. Surgeons will not jeopardize their own license by misrepresenting an insurance claim. If you run across a surgeon who makes a habit of recouping payment from insurance, you should run for the door. This is a dangerous and illegal practice that you should avoid at all cost. A reputable surgeon will usually know under which circumstances insurance can be billed. Neither you nor your surgeon should push the limit on this.

Although it may be tempting, do not be lured in by bargain rates or deep discounts. A physician should not have to market himself as the lowest priced surgeon in the area. Although the lowest price does not necessarily translate into the lowest quality, be wary of prices that are lower than the norm. Conversely, a higher price does not guarantee a better result. You may be paying for the luxurious office or new piece of technology. Quality and price often do not correlate—therefore, we do not recommend basing your decision strictly on price. If cost is an issue for you, feel free to discuss this with your physician or billing staff. There are surgeons who may be willing to negotiate their fees or arrange payment plans in certain circumstances.

If finances are an issue for you, there are some agencies that finance cosmetic surgery through a loan program. Your surgeon may be able to provide you with names of these agencies.

Are There Risks?

Of course there are risks. Make no mistake; even though cosmetic surgery is elective, there are still risks associated with it. As with any invasive procedure, the possible risks and complications must be reviewed and understood. There are obviously different risks inherent with each procedure. It is important in your consultation to openly discuss risks so that you can be fully informed when making your decision. Even experienced surgeons face complications, and you must accept that as a possibility when electing to have surgery. It is important for you to be fully apprised of all risks and complications associated with the procedure. We hope you don't change your mind after learning about the possible complications. Obviously, these complications are not expected outcomes. You surgeon has performed surgery many times and is well-aware of his or her complication rates. You can review the rates with your surgeon to put your mind at ease. Your job is to make a decision that the benefits outweigh the risks. We will provide more details about the risks for each procedure in their respective chapters.

Is There a Fee for Revisions?

A certain percentage of patients require a surgical revision. Some are a necessity due to an unexpected outcome. Others are performed simply because the patient is not 100% satisfied with the results. You don't want to anticipate a problem, but you should be prepared in the event that it happens. On occasion, the original surgery may create a deformity or asymmetry that does not disappear in the healing process. A revision may be necessary, but will usually not be performed until nine months after initial surgery. Operating too early may overcorrect the problem or create another one.

There is no set policy on how a surgeon deals with revisions. Some physicians perform revisions within the first year at no charge, some at reduced fees, and some at the full fee. Keep in mind that it is unusual for the facility or anesthesia fee to be reduced if you require a revision. Discuss with your surgeon how he or she would handle the possibility of a revision and all of the related fees.

Will I Pay for the Consultation?

The answer to this question is, "usually." Consultation fees range from zero to several hundred dollars. There is no standard practice for fees. Some physicians charge a nominal fee; some credit the consultation fee if you schedule the surgery. Some surgeons do offer free consultation as a marketing strategy, but probably add it to the surgical fee later on. Most surgeons do charge a consultation fee to cover the cost of the overhead and staff required to maintain an office. Consult fees also discourage too many "window shoppers" who make a habit of visiting surgeons, but never commit to surgery. Charging a reasonable consultation fee is considered normal practice as long as it is not exorbitant. When scheduling your appointment, it is wise to inquire about the consultation fee.

"I have consulted with a reputable surgeon, but he turned me down for surgery....why would that happen?"

The patient-surgeon relationship is built on mutual trust and communication. There are certain situations when a surgeon may elect not to perform surgery on a patient.

1. Patient wants perfection or has unrealistic expectations

2. Patient is seeking surgery for the wrong reasons

3. Patient's health status (physical or emotional) is too risky for surgery

4.   Patient wants a guaranteed outcome

5.   Patient requires the skills of a more specialized surgeon

6.   Patient will likely be non-compliant with post-operative instructions

7.   Patient is not able to commit the time for recovery

8.   Patient is a habitual shopper and jumps from surgeon to surgeon

9.   Patient and surgeon do not develop a rapport.

If your surgeon of choice does not accept you as a patient, our advice is not to take it personally. Speak to the surgeon and try to understand the reasons for the decision. What you hear may enlighten you as you move forward and meet other surgeons.

CHAPTER 4
Facilities, Fees, and Falling Asleep

One of the questions you will likely ask your surgeon is, "Where will I have my procedure?" Depending on your preference and that of your surgeon, you may have several options from which to choose. For some patients, privacy is their utmost concern; for others, cost will be a major deciding factor. There are generally three types of surgical facilities: the private physician's office, the outpatient surgery center, and the hospital-based surgical facility. Data from the American Society for Aesthetic Plastic Surgery indicates that 52% of total procedures are performed in an office facility, 25% in a hospital, and 23% in a free-standing outpatient surgery center. Each option has benefits and disadvantages that need to be considered when making your decision.

Physician's Private Office
Many physicians prefer to perform non-complex procedures in the comfort of their own office. These office-based facilities can range from simple operating rooms to the most sophisticated surgical suites which rival any hospital.

Benefits: This is usually the least expensive option since the overhead in an office is significantly lower than a larger facility or hospital. In addition, you usually do not have to pay separate facility and anesthesia fees (unless the surgeon employs an anesthesiologist). The employees are usually well-trained and familiar with the physician and his or her techniques. Staff members who always work together create a safer, more efficient process of care. Patients seeking a high degree of privacy often prefer to have their procedure in the physician's office. If there is only one surgeon performing surgery, patients are usually timed so that they do not bump into other patients. Physicians are usually more comfortable performing surgery in their offices since they are in control of the environment. Patients are usually very content having their procedures performed in their physician's office, but there are some drawbacks.

Disadvantages: Standardized regulations do not exist for a physician's private office. In many states, surgeons can perform procedures in their office without any credentialing or quality control processes. This lack of regulation can lead to an unqualified or untrained surgeon performing your surgery. Even though this is a worst case scenario, many are unaware of this possibility. We are not suggesting that there are always problems with all surgeons who perform procedures in their offices. There are many excellent, well trained surgeons who simply prefer to perform non-complex surgery in their office rather than an outpatient facility or hospital. If your surgeon suggests performing the procedure in the office, ask if he or she is also credentialed to perform the same procedure in the hospital. If the surgeon is credentialed, you can feel more secure that he or she has met the standards of the hospital, and is likely to be qualified and well-trained. If, however, the surgeon is not credentialed in any other facility, this should be regarded as a red flag.

The major disadvantage of a physician's office is the lack of back-up. This means that you are at greater risk if an untoward event or severe complication should occur. In a hospital, if you have a severe reaction to the anesthesia, there are highly trained personnel and high-tech equipment to immediately treat you. If necessary, you can be transported to the emergency room or intensive care unit. In some situations, this quick response can be the difference between life and death. In the office, it is likely that your surgeon does not deal with these emergencies too often. This factor may suggest that he or she is not the best person to deal with them such emergencies. They may not have the drugs or medications that are required. If such a problem did occur, it is likely that 911 would be called, which could result in treatment delays.

Ambulatory Surgery Center

These are usually free-standing centers that specialize in surgery and other outpatient procedures. An ambulatory surgery center may be affiliated with or operated by a hospital, or be privately owned. The typical ambulatory surgery center has several operating suites and ample waiting and recovery areas. They are usually nicely decorated and aesthetically pleasing to patients and their families.

Benefits: Some physicians prefer the ambulatory surgery center environment for their patients. Although the cost may be higher than that of a private office, it is usually well below that of hospitals. The overhead to operate an ambulatory center is lower than that of a hospital, which allows them to be more competitively priced. Usually, you will pay one global fee in an ambulatory surgery center that covers the operating room, supplies, anesthesia, equipment, and recovery room. This global fee, however, may not include the surgeon's fee, anesthesiologist fee, and pathologist's or assistant surgeon's fee.

The mission of these centers is to cater to the outpatient and make the process as smooth and pleasant as possible. The staff is specifically trained to provide outpatient care and have experience in expediting the entire process. Nurses and technical personnel are usually very familiar with the physicians and their procedures. The service and atmosphere may be perceived as more comfortable and patient friendly than a larger hospital setting. The aesthetics of the centers vary from the lavish, private havens to the more standard functional facility, but most are designed for the ambulatory patient. Ambulatory surgery centers are generally safer than a physician's private office if they have more sophisticated equipment and back-up systems.

Some states require ambulatory surgery centers to be accredited. Accreditation by a regulatory agency indicates that the care provided has met the strict standards set forth by that agency. The three main accreditation agencies are:
- American Association for Accreditation of Ambulatory Surgery Facilities
- American Association for Ambulatory Health Care
- Joint Commission on Accreditation of Healthcare Organizations

These organizations develop their own standards on staff, equipment, facilities, safety, and clinical care of patients. Facilities who elect to seek accreditation must demonstrate organizational compliance with these standards. You can investigate whether the facility used by your surgeon is accredited through the accrediting agency's website.

Disadvantages: Although generally considered safer than the average physician's office, this may or may not be true. An ambulatory surgery center may not have the hi-tech equipment and trained staff in the event that something goes wrong. In an event such as a heart attack, the personnel at the ambulatory surgery center may have to call 911, similar to a physician's office. There is a great deal of variation in the sophistication of these ambulatory facilities. They range from private storefront operations with no accreditation to the more sophisticated centers located within or proximate to major hospitals. Details about the facility should be reviewed with your physician.

If cost is a concern, keep in mind that fees in these centers are typically higher than those of a physician's office. You will need to weigh the cost against the benefits. Most ambulatory surgery centers offer a wide array of procedures and serve many patients on a given day. Due to the higher numbers of patients, this environment is not as private as a physician's office, but probably more discreet than a large hospital environment. The waiting and recovery areas will likely have other patients in them, creating more of a "hospital feel." In the recovery area, there may be less hand-holding (one on one care), as there are other patients who may require attention and or have emergencies.

Hospital-based Surgical Facility

Hospital-based surgery encompasses both ambulatory procedures and more complex surgeries that require an overnight stay or extended admission. For simple cosmetic procedures, even when having surgery at a hospital, the patient can go home on the same day of surgery. For more complicated surgery, an overnight stay may be necessary. Many hospitals have separate ambulatory waiting areas, operating rooms, and recovery areas that create a friendlier, less stressful experience for the patient and family.

Benefits: Hospitals are highly regulated organizations that must comply with numerous standards imposed by the State and Federal governments and accrediting agencies. Hospitals must comply with standards many agencies including:

- State Departments of Health
- Federal agencies such as the Center for Medicare Services
- Joint Commission for the Accreditation of Healthcare Organizations (JCAHO)

These standards cover areas such as patient safety, quality and environment of care, infection control, operating procedures, staff qualifications, and many more. There are also stringent regulations which address the credentialing process for physicians and other providers. Before a physician is permitted to operate in a hospital, he or she must be credentialed and granted privileges. These requirements are in place to ensure that the physicians possess the appropriate training, experience, and clinical competency to practice at the hospital. Hospitals must comply with regulations or else they run the risk of losing their accreditation and governmental and private insurance reimbursement.

Employees such as nurses, technicians, and assistants in a hospital are well-trained and must demonstrate on-going competency. In the event of an emergency, you will be treated immediately since there are highly skilled physicians and hi-tech equipment always available. Although no one can predict an emergency, the hospital is the safest place to be in the event that one occurs. Hospital employees are accustomed to dealing with these events, and receive on-going training to maintain their skills. You can easily be transported to a critical care unit or have medication administered if required.

Disadvantages: The most significant patient concerns about going to a hospital for surgery are the lack of privacy and increased cost. There will likely be other patients in the waiting areas, surgical areas, and recovery rooms. If you must stay overnight, there will be other patients on the floor or in your room. Many different staff members will be in and out of your room throughout your stay. There may be little private relaxation time in hospitals since they are usually noisy and busy, even throughout the night. If you are particularly concerned about keeping your surgery a secret, many hospitals offer private rooms or luxury suites at a premium rate that is paid out of pocket. Some hospitals will also allow you to register using an alias so that your name cannot be traced to that hospital. Many hospitals are accustomed to treating "VIPs" and will go to great lengths to protect your privacy.

Another disadvantage of the hospital stay is the cost. Since cosmetic surgery is typically out of pocket, you will be financially responsible for many items during the course of care. You will be billed for operating room time, medications, lab work, anesthesia, and supplies. If you stay overnight, you will have to pay a separate room charge. Some hospitals will have a discounted package rate for cosmetic procedures as an incentive. If you choose to stay overnight, the typical room charge is between $750 and $1200 per night. If you are permitted to leave after your procedure, you will save on the room charge but may need a private duty nurse. Hospital fees can be quite a bit higher than those of a free standing ambulatory surgery center or private surgeon's office because of the large overhead. You will likely be instructed that payment of fees is expected prior to or on the day of your surgery.

Fees: How Much Will My Surgery Cost?
The American Society for Aesthetic Plastic Surgery publishes annual data on Physician/Surgeon fees. These are average fees collected from a survey of physicians from across the country. It is important to note that there is significant variation by geographic region. States in the Northeast such as CT, MA, NH, NY, NJ, PA, and VT will command approximately 20-25% higher fees than the national average.

In addition to the surgeon's fee, remember that you will also be responsible for the facility fees. Some facilities will charge an hourly rate; others will have specific procedure fees. Some facilities will offer discounts if you pay the entire fee up front. If you can manage this, it is worth doing since it saves on cost. There may also be separately billed anesthesia fees, depending on the location. Fees are available on a number of websites from Plastic Surgery Associations and Societies. These lists of fees should only be used as a guide. Individual physician and facility fees will vary depending on whether the practice is in a rural, urban, or suburban area.

If your surgery involves an overnight hospital stay, you can plan on adding about $1000 per night to the facility fee. Additional costs such as implants (breast augmentations) or compression garments (Face lifts) will also be separately billable items. If two procedures are done on the same day, there may be a discounted rate for the second procedure. A detailed estimate of all costs should be reviewed with your physician or his office staff.

Falling Asleep: What type of Anesthesia Will Be Used?

There are three levels of anesthesia used in cosmetic surgery: local anesthesia, general anesthesia, and sedation anesthesia. Sometimes, they may be used in combination. At your consultation visit, the surgeon will usually make a recommendation regarding the preferred type of anesthesia for your case. You may have questions, concerns, or preferences of your own. Do not hesitate discussing these issues with the surgeon. For example, there are patients who prefer to be awake during surgery, and there are others who are fearful and want to be completely asleep. If you have had reactions to a particular type of anesthesia in the past, make sure you mention this as well. There are several options for "falling asleep." The more honest you are with your surgeon, the higher the likelihood that he or she will recommend the best option for you.

General and sedation anesthesia are usually administered by Anesthesiologists (physicians who have a minimum of three years of specialized training after medical school) or Nurse Anesthetists (nurses who have special training in anesthesia and work under the direction of the surgeon). Most surgeons usually have a preference about who they entrust to deliver anesthesia to their patients.

Local Anesthesia

Local anesthesia is the least complicated form of anesthesia and is usually given by the surgeon. Injection of a local anesthetic such as Lidocaine locally numbs an area of the body. Allergic reactions to local anesthesia are rare; it is considered to be the safest of all anesthesia options.

Unlike with general anesthesia, law does not require an anesthesiologist to be present when a patient receives local anesthesia. Patients are awake during their procedure so they are aware of the surgery, but do not feel discomfort. For particularly anxious patients, the surgeon may advise taking some Valium prior to the surgery. Some surgeons prefer Lidocaine combined with Epinephrine, which causes constriction of the blood vessels and reduced bleeding. Local anesthesia is commonly used in small procedures such as mole removal, fat injections, lip augmentation, Restylane® injections and upper blepharoplasty.

Sedation with Local Anesthesia

Sedation anesthesia is commonly referred to as "twilight" or monitored anesthesia care ("MAC"). Sedation involves the intravenous injection of medications to make you feel drowsy and relaxed. Even anxious patients will typically relax or fall asleep with sedation. Patients usually do not recall their procedure when they wake up. New medications leave the patient feeling refreshed rather than groggy and confused. Local anesthesia is often given in combination with sedation to reduce pain. Depending on the level of sedation, you may be totally asleep and unaware of the entire procedure, or only slightly drowsy.

You will breathe on your own with sedation, and do not need to be intubated (have a breathing tube inserted in your throat). Sedation is usually considered the best option by patients who do not want to be awake, but are afraid of general anesthesia. Sedation, however, has its own set of risks, which can be dangerous or even fatal if errors occur. There have been instances where patients become slightly agitated during the surgery, and the surgeon or anesthesiologist administers more anesthesia to create a deeper sedation. Deeper sedation can be a dangerous situation for patients. If a patient is overly sedated, he can become unresponsive and have difficulty breathing on his own. Unlike general anesthesia, where a patient's breathing is mechanically controlled, an over-sedated patient can run into problems. Although they are rare, there have been deaths associated with accidental over-sedation.

The safest way to avoid over-sedation is to have a board-certified anesthesiologist responsible for your sedation. Anesthesiologists have expertise in dosing and the levels of sedation, which improves safety and reduces the incidence of errors. When an attending anesthesiologist is present, it allows the surgeon to focus all of his or her attention on performing the surgery. This division of labor is the best situation, and one that we strongly recommend. There are some surgeons, however, who feel comfortable administering their own anesthesia. This option may be less expensive and attractive to some patients on a budget. The increased risk of not using an anesthesiologist should be weighed against the increased costs. In the end, you must be comfortable entrusting your surgeon with anesthesia in addition to tending to the details of your surgery. This is a discussion which you must have with your surgeon prior to your procedure. Sedation and local anesthesia are commonly used for Face lifts, liposuction, blepharoplasty, rhinoplasty, and breast augmentation.

General Anesthesia

General anesthesia is commonly used for longer, more complicated cosmetic procedures. High-tech monitoring equipment and newer, more advanced anesthetic agents have improved the safety and success of general anesthesia. There is little risk associated with general anesthesia since the environment is very controlled. Under general anesthesia, you will have a tube inserted in your airway to control your breathing mechanically. Drugs will be introduced intravenously, which will place you in an unconscious state. You will not feel any pain or recall any part of your surgery. Vital signs are monitored throughout the entire procedure by the anesthesiologist to ensure your safety. These safety controls allow the surgeon to focus all of his or her attention on the surgery. Local anesthesia is sometimes used in conjunction with general anesthesia to reduce pain and bleeding.

There is a misconception by many patients that general anesthesia is dangerous and should be avoided. This is a myth since the risks of this type of anesthesia are very low. Many patients have misinformation regarding anesthesia, which may cause fear or anxiety. We recommend that you become well-versed in the type of anesthesia you will receive and who will administer it. Often, you will meet the anesthesiologist immediately before your surgery, but this is not the time to engage in a lengthy discussion. Most often, the anesthesiologist will ask you a few questions and explain briefly what will occur. Detailed discussions on the benefits and risks of the various types of anesthesia should occur at your consultation with your surgeon. Most surgeons have years of experience and become comfortable with a small number of anesthesiologists and their techniques. This mutual trust that develops between physicians results in improved safety and the best outcome. General anesthesia is used for more complex surgeries such as breast reduction, breast augmentation, and abdominoplasty.

"I like my surgeon, but he is much more expensive than the others that I've met. I don't want to skimp on cost, but I don't want to overpay. What should I do? "

You should not make your decision primarily based on price, but you have to know what you are comparing. Did your surgeon include anesthesia and facilities fees in the quote? Are you certain that each physician quoted a fee for the same procedure? If there is a wide difference in price, ask the surgeon if he/she is doing the surgery himself and if he/she will be present for the entire time. Surgeons who perform the surgery and stay with you for the entire procedure may charge a higher fee.

Perhaps, the surgeon has specialized training and added expertise which produces finer work. Your surgeon may feel that his experience, training, or reputation commands a higher price. Overhead, geography, and reputation are all factors surgeons use to develop their own fee.

In the end, you have to be convinced that the higher fee is justified. Have an honest discussion with the physician. If you are still not comfortable, perhaps you should keep looking for another physician.

CHAPTER 5
How Should I Prepare For Surgery?

History and Physical

If you are over the age of 50, have any history of heart disease, diabetes, hypertension, pulmonary disease, or any significant medical history, you will be asked to see your internist for medical clearance. Even healthy patients who are over the age of 50 will likely need some medical clearance before surgery. In many cases, you may be asked to get a CBC (complete blood count), UA (urinalysis), PT and PTT (tests for coagulation), chest x-ray, and Electrocardiogram to get the full picture of your health status. This is routine operating procedure, so don't be alarmed if your surgeon asks for this clearance.

Make sure that you tell your surgeon of all prior surgeries you have had in the past. Many problems can be avoided or addressed if the surgeon has this information well in advance. The surgical technique or type of anesthesia may vary depending on the information you have provided to your surgeon. This is not the time to withhold any information from your surgeon.

Scheduling

Since cosmetic surgery is, for the most part, an elective procedure, you can schedule your procedure when it is most convenient for you and your surgeon. Ability to take time off, as well as season and temperature, may influence your decision. After some procedures, such as liposuction, you will need to wear compression garments that can be uncomfortable in the summer. In addition, you may be asked to avoid the sun following Face lifts or eye procedures. Although the total recovery time will vary by procedure, you should plan to be at home for one to two weeks after surgery. You should also plan for several follow-up appointments to your surgeon, so you will need to line up your transportation and someone to accompany you. You may also need to stay locally if you live far away from your surgeon's office.

Paying For Your Surgery

Now that you are fully aware of the fees from your consult visit, make sure that you know the timetable for payments. Some offices will not keep the reservation if all fees are not paid in advance. Each office may have different policies for payments, but most will expect payment up front. Make sure that you are prepared in the event that the operation takes longer than expected, or there are any additional procedures that you may desire. There is always a possibility that additional bills will crop up once you start on this journey. When planning your budget, it is wise to allot some unplanned expenses down the road. For example, it is common to have Collagen, Botox® procedures, lasering, or other non-invasive procedures to augment the surgical procedure. These additional procedures may not be estimated at the time of the surgery, but may be desired later on in the process. We wanted you to be aware that it is common to add other items down the road. If finances are an issue, you may want to plan ahead for these expenses. There are also companies which specialize in loans for cosmetic surgery. We cannot recommend any specific ones because they deal directly with the patient, but we are aware of patients who have received financing through this arrangement.

Medications

All patients who intend on having surgery must stop taking any medication that contains aspirin. Aspirin interferes with the clotting process and can cause bleeding problems in otherwise healthy patients. Some over-the-counter medications that may be beneficial to you for other symptoms can be harmful for surgical patients. Aspirin-containing products, and some non-steroidal anti-inflammatories and blood thinning agents will increase bleeding and complications. These need to be discontinued two weeks prior to surgery and not taken again until after two weeks post-surgery. If you are prescribed these medications by your internist, you must confer with your doctor before stopping them. You would be surprised how many over-the-counter medications contain aspirin or other blood thinning products. We have seen many patients who were taking medications containing aspirin and did not think it important enough to mention them to their surgeon. As a result, these medications were not discontinued, and the patient had unexpected bruising, bleeding, and other complications. It is extremely important that you list all medications for your surgeon, including over-the-counter medications which may seem harmless to you.

Below is a list of some common medications that should be temporarily discontinued before surgery. This is not an all-inclusive list, so check with your surgeon or pharmacist to see if your medication contains aspirin or aspirin-like products.

Advil	Four way Cold Tablets
Aleve	Furocet
Alka-Seltzer	Ibuprofen
Anacin	Indocin
Anaprox	Midol
Aspercreme	Motrin
Aspergum	Naprosyn
Bayer Aspirin	Norgesic
Bufferin	Nuprin
Cope	Pepto-Bismol
Coricidin	Percodan
Darvon	Sine-Aid
Doan's Pills	Sine-Off
Dristan	Triaminicin
Ecotrin	Vanquish
Excedrin	Vioxx
Fiorinal	Vitamin E
	Zomax

Alcohol

Alcohol consumption may increase the likelihood of bleeding and the development of a hematoma. It is recommended that you abstain from alcohol at least three days prior to your surgery.

Herbal Therapies

Herbal therapies are becoming very popular, but not viewed by some as medications. Therefore, many patients fail to tell their surgeons the herbal supplements that they are taking. There have not been enough studies on the effects of herbal therapies on surgery or anesthesia. Many surgeons will be cautious with herbal therapies and suggest discontinuing them two weeks prior to surgery. Below is a list of some herbal therapies that should be discontinued prior to surgery. Many of them may cause bleeding, rapid heart rate, high blood pressure, or decreased clotting if not discontinued prior to surgery.

Alfalfa
Caffeine Pills
Diet Pills containing Ephedra
Echinacea
Garlic pills
Ginger
Ginkgo Biloba
Ginseng

Goldenseal
Melatonin
St. John's Wort
Selenium

No Smoking!

Smokers have a higher incidence of complications which may lead to a less than satisfactory outcome. The nicotine in smoking causes small blood vessels to constrict which decreases the blood flow and the ability of the body to heal. Decreased blood flow may cause the skin to turn black and die (skin necrosis). It is essential that smoking be stopped at least two weeks prior to surgery and two weeks afterwards. Perhaps this cosmetic surgery and a new outlook on life is exactly what you need to permanently quit smoking! Your surgeon may be able to provide you with a smoking cessation program or a nicotine patch to get you on your way toward a healthier lifestyle.

Supplements to Aide Healing

There are some supplements that you should begin taking prior to your surgery to decrease bruising. These are not absolutely necessary, but many people can benefit from this extra help.

Vitamin K (also known as mephyton) helps clotting and reduces bruising. Vitamin K is a key component in the blood clotting process.

Typically, you will be prescribed 5 mg once per day beginning five days before surgery.

Vitamin C helps the healing process and may reduce bruising. We recommend 500 mg three times a day.

Bromelain is an active ingredient found in fresh pineapple and has been found to help decrease swelling and bruising. You can purchase Bromelain in tablet form in vitamin shops and you should take 500 mg three times a day. Or, you can eat two slices of fresh pineapple once a day for five days before surgery.

Arnica is a homeopathic medication used in China for centuries. It comes in pill form and topical cream. The cream can be used post-operatively, but more importantly, take a pill on the morning of surgery with one small sip of water.

What You Will Need To Purchase

You will not be able to go shopping for last minute items after your surgery so you should stock up well in advance. In addition to the supplies below, you may want to go grocery shopping before your surgery and have some meals prepared, or have some take out menus available. The last thing you will want to hear when you get home is, "Hey, mom, what's for dinner?"

Here are some supplies that you should have on hand when you get home.

- Pain medication prescription should be filled and sitting on your nightstand. Take the medication as directed. This is not the time to be a martyr. The surgeon gave you pain medication for several reasons. By decreasing the discomfort, this helps to reduce your blood pressure and heart rate. High levels of pain will increase heart rate and blood pressure, which can complicate the healing process. After three days of taking pain medication, you may able to switch to Tylenol if you feel that it is strong enough to control your pain.

- Stool Softener for constipation that may occur as a result of taking pain medication
- Any antibiotics that may have been prescribed, as well as a prescription for vaginal yeast infections if you are prone to these when taking antibiotics
- A cooler with ice to make cold compresses. Cool compresses are a must. We are not prescriptive about what kind; you can try them all and see which you prefer. You can use moistened gauze pads, plastic bags with crushed ice, commercial ice packs, or frozen vegetables. The cold packs should be applied for ten minutes, removed for ten minutes, and so on for the first 48 hours
- Benedryl (over the counter) in case of itching or to aide sleeping
- Baby shampoo
- Gentle, non-fragranced soap (Dove or Ivory)
- Gauze pads and tape
- Extra pillows to prop you upright
- Keep glasses handy if you usually wear contacts

Plan for Some Extra Help

Some patients and physicians prefer to use a private duty nurse for the first night after surgery. The nurse will obtain most of the supplies, apply your cold packs, administer your medication, get you some food or drink, look for signs of complications, and communicate with your surgeon if necessary. The average fee for a private duty nurse can range between $500 and $1000, but it is well worth the money if you can afford it. If not, make sure you line up a friend or family member who can stay with you during the night and perform these functions.

Hair Coloring and Perms

If you are having surgery on your face, and you color or perm your hair, it is recommended that you do this prior to your surgery. For many weeks, your skin and scalp will be tender and cannot be exposed to chemicals such as hair dyes or perms.

Limit Guests and Activity

After a few days, when you begin to feel better, you will have the urge to show off your surgery. Resist this urge and do not invite friends or family over to see the new you. Remember that you have had a surgical procedure and rest is essential to assist in the healing process. Over-activity can cause bleeding or other complications. Even if you are feeling well, make an effort to rest. If you are able, you may watch television, DVDs, or read a magazine. This is not the time to catch up on errands or rearrange your closets. Preserve this healing time for yourself; there will be plenty of time to show off in the future.

CHAPTER 6
How to Survive the Day of Surgery

The day of surgery has finally arrived. It has probably been weeks or months since you had made your decision and selected your surgeon. You have done your research, interviewed your surgeon, decided on your procedure, and paid your fees. Now it is time to go through with the surgery.

How Do You Feel?

On the morning of surgery, you will probably be somewhat nervous, but excited with anticipation. Some people become very anxious and start to question their decision. There are common concerns and questions that arise at this late stage of the game. If you are feeling or thinking any of these, you are not alone.

- Should I really be doing this?
- Am I doing the right thing?
- Will I feel any pain?
- Will I be happy with my result?
- What if I don't wake up from anesthesia?
- What if I bleed or get an infection?
- Is this surgery worth the risks that were listed on the consent?

These questions are a normal part of gearing up for the surgery. You will likely tell yourself that it is time to trust both your instincts and your surgeon's skills and move ahead. If, however, you have major concerns, feel panicky, or seriously think you are making a mistake, you should speak with your surgeon immediately. You always have the right to change your mind and cancel the procedure. Remember that on the morning of surgery, you should be able to speak with your physician to review the plan. It is likely that your surgeon will see you briefly and make some markings on your skin. These few moments before surgery are very helpful for both you and the surgeon. You should never be put to sleep without fist seeing your surgeon to verify consent and procedure.

On the Morning of Surgery

There are a few basic ground rules to follow when going for surgery. These will usually apply irrespective of the location of your surgery.

- Do not eat or drink anything after midnight
- If you take medication, follow your surgeon's instructions about whether to take them or skip a dose
- Arrive on time to the facility or office
- Leave jewelry and valuables at home
- Do not bring a lot of cash with you
- Wear loose fitting clothing
- If you are having face or eye surgery, wear a front-opening top so you do not have to pull it over your head
- Make sure that you have someone lined up to take you home after surgery
- Take the phone number of your pharmacy in case the surgeon needs to call in any prescriptions
- Take all insurance cards with you
- Fill all prescriptions ahead of time so that you have them ready after surgery
- Double check all supplies if you are returning home after surgery

It's Time!

You will be given a time to arrive at the facility or office which may be one to two hours prior to your actual surgery time. Please ensure that you are not late because you will be kept busy while waiting for your surgery to begin. This is the time for completion of paperwork, interviews by the nurse, and those final words with the surgeon or anesthesiologist. It is also possible that the earlier surgeries will be quicker than expected, or even cancelled, enabling you to be called in earlier.

When you arrive at the facility or surgeon's office, you will likely be greeted by a receptionist who will be expecting you. You will change into a gown and place your belongings in a locker or changing room. A nurse will meet with you, perhaps ask for a brief history, take your vital signs, and ask last minute questions. If you are not feeling well, perhaps have a cold or cough, you should advise the nurse. Surgery may be postponed if you are not feeling well to avoid complications or risks. You will then be led into a holding area or pre-op room. You may meet the anesthesiologist and answer some questions. It is here that you may be sedated and prepared for surgery. Once the surgeon and team are ready, you will go to the operating room. The operating room will look very intimidating and sterile, and you may get nervous walking into the room. This is completely normal; before you know it, people will be busy all around you. Each person on the team has a role in delivering the best possible care to you. You will have some monitoring equipment hooked up to measure heart rate, blood pressure, and oxygen saturation. If not already done in the pre-op room, you will have an intravenous (IV) line started so that anesthesia can be administered. Once the surgeon and anesthesiologist are ready, you are now on your way to becoming more beautiful.

Waking Up

When you wake up, you will probably be in the recovery room. You will not remember having the surgery, but will notice dressing, wrapping, or some other indication of what has just happened. You will want to look in a mirror immediately, but will have to wait a little while. If you had general anesthesia, you may experience a dry or sore throat from the tube that was inserted. Some patients experience nausea or vomiting, which will subside or be treated with medication. You may still feel groggy or weak and just want to nap during the time in the recovery area. The nurse may give you ice chips, liquids, or a small snack prior to going home. Depending on the procedure, you will spend at least an hour or two in the recovery area before being permitted to leave. Once you are ready for discharge, you will be given post-op instructions and any additional prescriptions that you may need. You will also be told when to make your follow-up appointment with the surgeon. In many cases, this appointment is the next day, so make sure that you pay attention to this timetable. Someone will have to drive you home because it will be a while before you are able to drive yourself. You can now leave to begin your road to recovery!

Recovery Period

Be prepared; the next few days will be an emotional roller coaster ride. You will likely be very tired during the first 24-72 hours. When you start to get around and look in the mirror, you will notice bruising and swelling. You will probably be asking yourself why you did this to yourself. You may even have some anger or resentment. Over the next day or two, there is more bruising and you are thinking that the surgery was a huge mistake. The surgeon did warn you that the swelling and bruising would look worse before it looks better, but it is still upsetting. These feelings of doubt and concern are completely normal.

On day three, you will feel less lethargic and able to get around the house. There is still a good deal of bruising and swelling and you may still not be able to see your improvement. On day four, you will notice that the swelling subsides, and the bruising is not getting any worse. You are finally thinking that the tides are turning, and this may all be fine. You may even see a glimmer of improvement as you look into the mirror. Over the week, the bruising subsides significantly and you are convinced that you've made the right decision. By now, you have already seen your surgeon and he or she has reassured you that you are progressing nicely.

At week one or two, you will likely return to work or your regular activities. You may be a bit self-conscious. You will have to decide whether or not to disclose to people that you have had cosmetic surgery. Friends and relatives will be your support system as you regain normalcy. At six weeks, you will feel better and something miraculous happens. Everything feels and looks better and the improvements are more noticeable. You regain your self-confidence and feel great. You will start to recommend cosmetic surgery to your skeptical family and friends. You may even wonder what else you can do for yourself next year!

PART II
Surgical Procedures

There are many different cosmetic surgery procedures. Listed below are the most common procedures. Each chapter will include information on pain scale, length of procedure in time, time required before resuming normal activities, description of procedure and recovery. Also included are some Do's and Don'ts as well as complications which may have been associated with the procedure.

This is not an all-inclusive list of procedures. There are many others which are performed but this is representative of the common procedures performed in the United States in 2006.

CHAPTER 7
The Face Lift (Rhytidectomy)

Pain scale: 5 out of 10
Length of Procedure: 3 to 4 hours
Back To Work Time: 2 weeks

A face lift (also known as Rhytidectomy) encompasses several types of procedures that lift the cheeks, jowls, and neck areas. Most face lifts involve the following procedures:

- Removal of excess skin on the face
- Tightening of skin and tissues under the skin
- Removal of excess skin under the neck
- Tightening of the neck muscle
- Removal of jowls or fat under the neck

The combination of any or all of these procedures may be performed depending on the desired outcome. A typical candidate for a face lift is usually someone in their forties to seventies who has skin hanging from their neck, face, and jowls. During a Face lift, excess skin is removed and the muscles tightened to create the "lift" and eliminate sagging. Excess fat is then liposculpted, which is similar to liposuction. A Face lift will not greatly impact the nasolabial folds or creases that run from your nose to both sides of your mouth. To treat these creases, you may require fillers (such as Collagen or Restylane) or laser treatments months after the surgery. If a face lift is done well, you will have a more youthful look with no telltale signs of surgery. If your surgeon is skilled, your new face should appear youthful and natural without looking taut or pulled.

Procedure
The procedure is usually done under light sedation (MAC anesthesia). Once the patient is comfortable, local anesthetic is injected at the site.

Incisions are strategically placed to hide the most visible scars behind the ears and in the hair. Typically, incisions are placed in the hair above the ear, and others placed in front of the ear or hidden inside. If necessary, the jowl area may be liposculpted to eliminate excess fat. (Note that this fat may be used later as natural filler much like Collagen) The skin is lifted back into position on your face, creating a more youthful look. A skillful surgeon will suture skin back in a meticulous manner so that scarring is minimal. Incisions that are in front of the ear will heal very well over time and not be noticeable. The skin that is lifted is supported mainly by sutures placed behind the ear. This area is subjected to the greatest pull or tension, which typically leads to some visible scarring. Since the hair is not shaved, incisions are delicately made in between follicles, which help to camouflage them. The surgeon must also work very carefully to avoid traumatizing the nerves to reduce the risk of permanent numbness. If looking closely at this area, your hairdresser will know that you had surgery, but no one else.

The procedure usually requires three to four hours. At the end of the procedure, your surgeon will apply a helmet-like dressing around your face. Some surgeons apply drain tubes in the neck area for a 24 hour period. The purpose of the drain is to collect excess fluid in a neat way. If a drain is not placed, expect staining on the back of your dressing. This staining is completely normal and no cause for alarm. Some surgeons do not use drains because they are concerned that small track marks are left under the skin, which is a telltale sign of surgery.

Different Types of Face lifts

With all of the television shows and media hype recently, you may have heard about a variety of Face lift procedures. Different surgeons use different techniques to achieve the desired outcome. There is no right or wrong technique. Your surgeon will choose the correct procedure based on your desired results and his or her surgical preference. As a patient, you should be made aware of the advantages and disadvantages of each approach. You are not expected to understand the technical details of each procedure, just the overall plan.

Dialing the clock back and making you appear more youthful and rested is the goal. After a Face lift, you should look refreshed and rejuvenated, not like a totally different person. The best way to achieve this outcome is to use multiple layers to secure the Face lift. Some patients and surgeons believe that a more dramatic look is preferable. There are some celebrities (you know who they are!) who look overdone or stretched too tight. This look may be appropriate for them and exactly what they wanted. But for most people, that overdone look is not the desired outcome. We will now enumerate some techniques that are commonly used to by surgeons to perform Face lifts. This description will give you broad categories providing a frame of reference. The exact names and specific techniques of the procedures may vary by surgeon.

Skin Face lift: This procedure involves lifting only one layer of skin, excising the excess, and suturing the remaining skin into the proper position. The advantage of this procedure is that it's the simplest Face lift performed and has the lowest risk of nerve damage. This procedure is commonly referred to as the Mini-lift. One possible disadvantage of this procedure is a widening of scars over time due to lack of support from underneath. This Face lift may also not stand the test of time and need to be redone in a few years.

Two Layer Face lift: This two layer technique, also called the SMAS Face lift, is one of the most common. This procedure involves the skin and a deeper, tougher layer beneath, which is used as a support system. The subcutaneous musculo-aponeurotic substance (SMAS) is a strong supportive layer in the face. In the neck, the second supportive layer is a muscle called the platysma. This two layered technique adds longevity to the Face lift and reduces tension on the skin. In this procedure, each layer (SMAS and platysma) is tightened and lifted independently of one another. The advantages of this procedure are finer scar lines that heal nicely, longer lasting results and improvement in the mid-face area. The disadvantage is that it requires more surgical skill. You may also have some swelling from sutures which subsides over time. Many surgeons consider this procedure the ideal balance of safety and results.

Deep Plane Face lift: This procedure is also referred to as the subperiosteal Face lift. This surgical approach is quite extensive and produces a more dramatic result. In this procedure, all structures including skin, SMAS, muscles, and deep layers on the bones are moved to new positions. This movement of all layers causes the most drastic change, but can cause extended swelling. Some surgeons dissect deep into the nerves, but this has been associated with an increased nerve weakness after surgery. The advantage of this technique is that it creates a dramatic difference in appearance for those who want it. The skin will look tighter and more pulled than in the other procedures. There is also more swelling and bruising associated with this procedure. This procedure should be reserved for those who insist on a major change because the increased risk must be weighed against the outcome.

Post-operative Recovery Period
Day One

Most patients can go home a few hours after the procedure. Some opt to stay close by, at a hospital or hotel with a family member or private duty nurse. For the first evening, and overnight, it is important to apply cool compresses to the facial area that is exposed to reduce bruising and swelling. Elevation is also important so you will need two pillows under your head to decrease swelling. Keep the lights dim and try to rest for the first evening. There is some discomfort and pulling associated with a Face lift that can be well managed with medication. During this first evening, you will feel pressure or tightness in your neck area; this is normal and will dissipate over the next six week period. The suppleness in the neck will also return over the next few weeks. You should limit your activity except for applying the cold compresses and walking to the bathroom. You may feel some discomfort, but not sharp or shooting pain. Patients always state that they are actually surprised by the lack of pain with this procedure. Many patients fearful that there is a great deal of pain associated with face lifts, but this fear is unwarranted. One reason for this lack of pain is that nerve endings for sensation have been cut during the procedure. They will grow back in a few months and cause no permanent damage. When you look in the mirror, you may find that your smile is not symmetrical, which can be distressing. This asymmetry is due to muscle weakness as a result of anesthesia. Do not panic; as the local anesthesia continues to wear off and the nerves wake up, the muscles will return to normal function.

Many patients utilize the services of a private duty nurse. While this service may seem luxurious, it brings great benefit that will improve your recovery period. The nurse will apply the cold compresses, administer pain medication, tend to your needs, and help you through the initial recovery period. She will also function as a watchful eye overnight. A private duty nurse is experienced and will be looking for small signs of impending complications. If any are noticed, she will notify your surgeon immediately. For example, if you experience a sudden onset of intense pain, especially on only one side of your neck, associated with increased swelling, your physician should be notified. He or she will check for a hematoma, which is a collection of blood under the skin. A hematoma requires medical attention within a few hours, so immediate detection is valuable.

There is a very predictable pattern of emotions that occur with this procedure in most patients. While not everyone goes through the same phases on the same day, the similarity of emotions is quite remarkable. The best analogy for this pattern is a roller coaster ride. The next morning, the drop on the roller coaster ride begins! You have made it all the way up the mountain, you did your research, you had your surgery, you survived the night, and now you are asking "Why On Earth Did I Do This?" You will be swollen, look bruised, and in some discomfort. You are starting to question your decision about the surgery. This emotional reaction is quite normal and expected. After you go to your surgeon for your post—op visit, you will have your dressing removed and your face will be checked. After this visit, you will feel much more comfortable and reassured.

Days Two and Three
Over the next 48-72 hours, you will see more swelling and bruising in all areas of your face. The amount of bruising will vary by individual but will be at its worst on day three. Patients should always be prepared to expect this increase in swelling and bruising until day three. There will be some discomfort because you cannot easily move your head and neck due to swelling. At this point, you will likely have looked at yourself in the mirror. You will notice that the jowls and fat are gone and there is a change in the shape of your face! You start to feel that there is light at the end of the tunnel. The emotional roller coaster is starting to climb to a better place. On the second day after surgery, you can get into a warm shower with gentle soap. You will look forward to washing your hair because it has become matted and caked with dried blood. A light stream of water and baby shampoo will work wonders and you will feel human again. You will have numbness around the face and ears that gradually improves over the next few months. You should be proud of yourself; the worst is now behind you.

Days Five to Seven

Your doctor will remove the fine sutures in front of your ear in the first week. By now, some of the bruising has started to subside, and you will see a yellowish color rather than the previous black or purple. Also, the swelling may be reduced enabling you to turn your head and neck more easily. You can now sleep on your sides and will likely be more comfortable. You are beginning to feel much better and may start to use make-up. Every day, you will look better and better, with incremental improvements occurring over the next several weeks. At this point, you start to believe that this could be a good thing and you look forward to seeing the final result.

Weeks Two to Six

With cover-up makeup you will be able to return to your normal routine. The emotions are generally positive and you feel pleased that you had the surgery. You still should refrain from strenuous activity until a full six weeks have elapsed. Over the next several weeks, there will be a few issues that will worry you such as numbness of earlobes, continued swelling, asymmetries, itching behind the ears, and crusty blood in the ears. You may be concerned about these and see your surgeon. He or she is likely to advise that these side-effects are normal and you should not be alarmed. At two weeks, you may resume some physical activity such as walking fast, light weights (five lbs) or stationary bike. Do not attempt anything too stressful or strenuous. If you feel comfortable, you may return to work in 14 days. Major social engagements where you will be the focus of attention should be avoided for six weeks. After six weeks, you can usually return to your normal activities.

Months later, the emotional roller coaster will be a fond memory and you will love your new youthful appearance. You will likely ask yourself, "Why didn't I do this sooner?" Your friends and family will be amazed and start to express their own interest in pursuing surgery. Typically, the "friends" that discouraged you before will be the first in line to have surgery after seeing your results.

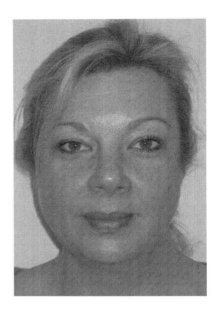

Face lift Front Pre-op

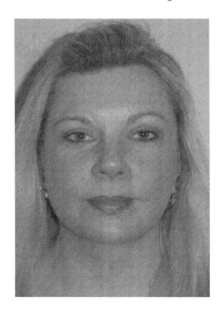

Face lift Front Post-op

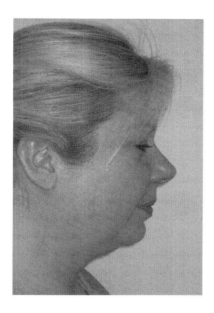

Face lift Side Pre-op

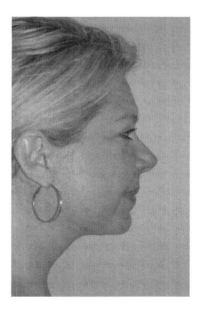

Face lift Side Post-op

Do's and Don'ts

- Don't attempt to clean your incisions with alcohol or astringents. This will cause them to become irritated and heal poorly
- Do wash with gentle soaps
- Don't plan to catch up on errands during your first few days after surgery
- Don't color your hair for six weeks after surgery
- Don't blow dry your hair on a hot setting for at least six weeks while the skin heals
- Don't succumb to advertisements. You will see many ads that tout the weekend face lift. This commonly refers to liposuction to remove fat from under the chin but does not remove the excess skin. Remember, if the surgery is minimal, the change will be modest. The only way to eliminate hanging, excess skin is to excise it. This requires a full Face lift with a two week recovery period. Anything else should be researched thoroughly to ascertain the pros and cons

"How Long Will My Face lift Last?"

Everyone considering a face lift asks this question, but there is not an easy answer. The number of years a face lift will last depends on a variety of factors: age, sun damage, type of procedure performed, skin type, and patient expectation. The skin that is excised is gone forever, but this does not halt the aging process. Typically, the skin can continue to tighten for up to nine months after the surgery.

Unfortunately, gravity and nature start the clock ticking all over again. So what does this all really mean? When a 55 year old has a face lift, they typically shave ten years off their face. Their new 45 year old appearance may continue to look wonderful for 10 years. As the years progress, however, they will no longer have the face of a 45 year old. The skin will continue to age and sag over the course of many years. Some patients who have their first face lift in their 40s may find it desirable to have another procedure in their 50s or 60s. Others, however, will allow nature to take its course. Patients having their first face lift in their 60s may be more willing to accept some sagging skin in their 70s because this is age appropriate. Our advice is to make your decision based on the facts available to you here and now. Do not base your decision heavily on whether or not you will repeat the surgery in the future.

Possible Complications

Listed below are some possible complications that may occur with this procedure. Your surgeon will review the possible complications with you when you are asked to consent for surgery.

- **Bleeding:** It is possible, though unusual, that excessive bleeding may occur during or after surgery. Should post-operative bleeding occur, it may require emergency treatment to drain accumulated blood. Accumulations of blood under the skin (hematoma) may delay healing.
- **Scarring:** Many of the wounds will heal well with no visible or permanent scarring. Abnormal scars may sometimes occur within the skin and deeper tissues. Scars may be unattractive and of different color than the surrounding skin. There is also the possibility of visible marks from sutures.
- **Infection:** Infections are not common but may occur after any type of surgery. Antibiotic treatment or additional surgery may be necessary.
- **Nerve or Tissue Damage:** Deeper structures such as blood vessels, muscles, and particularly nerves may be damaged during the course of surgery. The potential for this to occur varies with the type of Face lift procedure performed. Injury to deeper structures may be temporary or permanent. Weakness, loss of facial sensation, or movement may occur after Face lift surgery, but should improve over time.

CHAPTER 8
Nose Job (Rhinoplasty)

Pain Scale: Complete	7 out of 10
Pain Scale: Tip only	3 out of 10
Length of Procedure:	1-2 hours
Return To Work:	1 week

Arhinoplasty is a procedure that alters the shape of the nose, Over 200,000 rhinoplasties were performed in 2005 as reported by the ASPS data. It is one of the most common cosmetic procedures as it has great impact on facial aesthetics. Rhinoplasty is one of the most technically demanding surgical procedures. Some surgeons with particular expertise have focused their practice primarily on rhinoplasty. You should seek out a surgeon who has expertise in the nasal area because specialized training and expertise in rhinoplasty will lead to optimal results. Like fashion trends, this surgery has gone through changes in techniques and outcome. Currently, a natural looking nose that fits with your facial features is the best result. The best compliment that someone can give you after a nose job is that you look great, but they don't know why. It was common in the 1970s for young women to flock to surgeons to get ski sloped noses or pinched tipped noses. This artificial and overdone look is now frowned upon and a more natural look is what most people want. Many of these women later seek revision surgery to improve nasal airway breathing and to eliminate the artificial look which resulted over the years of healing.

What is meant by years of healing? Of all the procedures, the rhinoplasty takes the longest time to see the final results. While major bumps that are removed can be seen immediately, the final sculpted shape will not be visible for at least a year. This is often difficult for patients to fully accept and understand. The nose may be sculpted down, but it also swells more than other parts of the body. If a finesse sculpting has been done on the tip, the swelling will overshadow the new shape that lies beneath. Over months, the swelling subsides and the natural sculpting that was performed will become visible. When it was more common to over sculpt, the results would look good after surgery, but in the ensuing years, the nose would get deformed. With nose jobs, unfortunately, there are no shortcuts. A patient's comprehension and acceptance of this transition time is critical for long term success.

Procedure

This is typically done under general anesthesia, but in selected cases, it may be done with sedation and local anesthesia. This procedure is usually performed on an outpatient basis and requires only one to two hours. There are two different types of rhinoplasties; closed and open.

In a closed rhinoplasty, all incisions are made inside the nose and there are no external visible incisions. This is remarkable—it is like working on a car from underneath without lifting the hood. An open approach requires an incision at the nasal tip (columella). Many patients are fearful of this external incision, however, over months, this heals very well. No one will easily detect this scar. Your surgeon may advocate for this procedure if he needs to get better exposure of the nose. This is sometimes needed when grafting is required or more sculpting is necessary. In an open procedure, there may be more swelling, but it should not deter you from moving ahead with this technique if your surgeon suggests it.

In either approach, the surgeon sculpts the framework (cartilage) that gives the new shape of the nose. The skin shrinks down to the new underlying shape. The top portion, which is mostly bony, is polished with an emory board type device. The polishing removes any bumps or irregularities in the nose. The final step involves, when necessary, breaking the bones and narrowing the bridge of the nose. At the end of the procedure, your surgeon will elect to hold everything in position using several techniques. Most commonly, a plastic nasal splint will be placed on the nose to keep the bones in proper alignment. A drip pad will be placed under your nose to collect blood. You may need to change the drip pad, but do not attempt to remove or alter the splint. A small cotton plug with a black string is inserted into the nose to collect any dripping blood. The dripping of blood is expected and should not be alarming. Some surgeons also use packing in the nose which is a long piece of gauze to help hold things in position.

Day One: Post-operative Recovery Period

You will be waking up in the recovery room and you will notice that your throat is scratchy and dry. You will notice some blood dripping down your lip or some blood tinged saliva. Do not be alarmed, this is to be expected. You can expect bruising and swelling to occur around the surgical areas. There will be black and blue marks under your eyes which are unsightly but will resolve gradually over the next 2-4 weeks. You may not have much discomfort at this point because the local anesthetic is still numbing the area. Cool compresses should be applied to the cheek areas for the next 48 hours. Frozen peas also work well because they can conform to the contours of your face. You can also use water with ice cubes placed in a washcloth. Bring extra tissues and gauze for the car ride home to catch some dripping blood. You should also wear old clothing since it may get blood stained and shirts which button down the front. Do not wear sweaters that pull over your head. That evening, you will feel the local anesthesia wearing off and you may feel discomfort in the bones of your nose. This is the time to take your pain medication as prescribed. If antibiotics were prescribed, you can start to take them the next morning after surgery. Rest with your head elevated on two pillows and continue with the cool compresses. You may not shower until the splint is removed. If you did shower, it would dislodge the splint. The water will dissolve the glue that is holding the splint and this will remove the necessary protection from your nose. You should try and rest for the first 24 hours after surgery.

For the first 72 hours, you should expect to see more swelling and bruising. This is completely normal and will subside by day 4.

Weeks One and Two

The next morning, you may pull the little black string that is taped to your nose and slide the cotton out. There will be a trickling of blood and you may get a breath of air, which will be a relief. Your nose will be congested similar to a head cold and this congestion may last up to six weeks. During this time period, you may spray 4 squirts of nasal saline solution into your nostrils every hour to help dissolve any dried blood. The more you do this, the better you will feel. Nasal saline can be bought over the counter in any pharmacy. You may also take Neosporin on a cotton swab and gently place it at the tip of your nostrils three times per day. The lubrication from the spray and the cream will moisturize the nasal lining and help to reduce the crusting. Usually, in the first week, the splint and any stitches will be removed. Your nose will look swollen and you will have bruising around your eyes if your bones have been moved. The bruising can be covered up with make-up. Many department stores carry customized concealers which blend in with your skin and cover bruising. Although the swelling will last several weeks, the bruising will resolve in about a week to ten days. In two weeks, you can start to do low impact aerobic exercises. Do not participate in strenuous activities or ones in which you could get injured.

Six Weeks On

In six weeks, you can resume all normal activities. By now, the bones have re-healed and the tenderness has resolved. The tip of your nose feels numb, woody, and hard, which is normal. Over the course of several months to a year, the pliability and softness will return. The soft contours and curves of your new nose will be defined and you can fully appreciate your new shape.

It is important to understand that the body does not heal symmetrically. In Nature, when there is healing and bruising, it is typically uneven and not perfectly symmetrical for some period of time. Over time, it all evens out but you will need to wait a full year to see the final result.

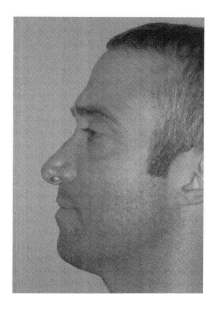

Rhinoplasty side pre-op

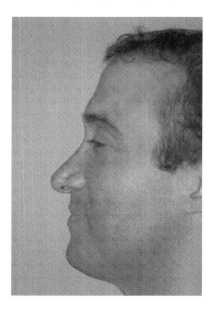

Rhinoplasty side post-op

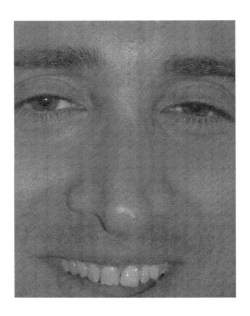

Rhinoplasty front pre-op

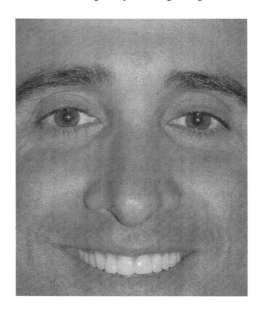

Rhinoplasty front post-op

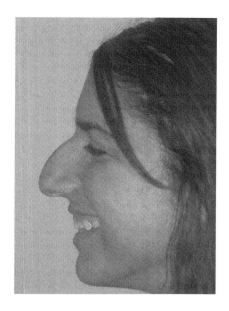

Rhinoplasty side pre-op

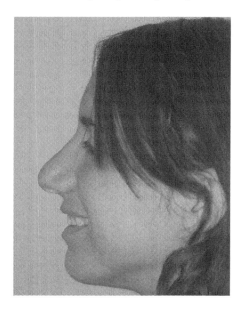

Rhinoplasty side post-op

Dos and Don'ts

- Do be careful picking up children, since young kids can hit your nose
- Don't engage in rough playing or playing with dogs for six weeks
- Don't exercise too early as it may increase swelling
- Do call your physician if the blood is dripping out of your nose excessively or if you have a fever greater than 102 degrees
- Don't panic if the nose just doesn't look right for a while; it takes a full year for final result
- Don't get sunburned for the first twelve months—you should wear a hat and suntan lotion with spf 30 or greater
- Don't pick your nose as it may cause bleeding and interfere with the healing process
- Do sleep on your back whenever possible
- Don't fly for two weeks following surgery. All of the swelling in the back of your nose and ears will have subsided by then making it more comfortable to fly
- Do ask your surgeon if you can use tape on your nose at night to help reduce swelling.

Possible Complications

Listed below are some possible complications that may occur with this procedure. Your surgeon will review the possible complications with you when you are asked to consent for surgery.

- **Bleeding:** Excessive bleeding may require emergency treatment.
- **Infection:** Infection is very rare unless some synthetic material is placed inside the nose. If an implant is being placed, your surgeon would have reviewed this with you and would have required your consent prior to surgery.
- **Unanticipated results:** There is the possibility of an unanticipated result from the rhinoplasty surgery. The surgery may result in unacceptable visible deformities, loss of functionality, or structural problems. Occasionally, you may be disappointed if the outcome of the rhinoplasty surgery does not

meet your expectations. Additional surgery may be necessary should the final result of rhinoplasty be unsatisfactory.

- **Numbness:** Although not common or predictable, there is the potential for permanent numbness within the nasal skin after rhinoplasty. Loss of skin sensation in the nasal area may not totally resolve over time.
- **Perforation:** Although very rare, there is a possibility that the rhinoplasty will cause a hole in the nasal septum. If this does occur, additional surgical treatment may be necessary to repair the hole in the septum.
- **Nasal airway alterations:** Changes may occur after a rhinoplasty that may interfere with normal nasal breathing.

CHAPTER 9
Tummy Tuck (Abdominoplasty)

Pain scale: 8 out of 10
Length of Procedure: 2 to 3 hours
Return To Work Time: 2 to 3 weeks

A tummy tuck (abdominoplasty) is a procedure that tightens the abdominal muscles and eliminates excess skin to create a smoother, flatter look. There are different types of tummy tucks. A full abdominoplasty must be differentiated from a mini-tummy tuck or liposuction of the belly. Patients seeking a tummy tuck usually have stable weights, but have excess skin that does not contract after liposuction. Sometimes, the muscles may be weak or spread apart from several pregnancies. Dieting and exercise have not been effective and the patient feels that surgical intervention is necessary to regain their youthful shape.

Unlike several of the other cosmetic procedures, a tummy tuck is very uncomfortable (this is what surgeons say when they really mean painful!) You should prepare for a long recovery period, since it takes almost two weeks before you can even stand upright. A tummy tuck is often coupled with liposuction of the flanks (sides of the abdomen) to create as trim a look as possible.

Tummy Tuck or Liposuction?
Liposuction reduces excess fat but will not eliminate sagging skin or loosened muscles. If you have what you consider excess fat, but your muscles and skin are tight, you may get your desired results from liposuction. However, if you have excess skin and weakened muscles, liposuction alone may not be the answer. Liposuction has the advantage of minimal scarring and an easier recovery. In some selected cases, the results are great. The disadvantage is that it takes months to see the final

changes and even after it is healed, the skin may feel irregular. After examining you, your surgeon will recommend the best procedure.

Procedure

Abdominoplasty is performed under general anesthesia. An incision is usually made at the bottom of the tummy from hip to hip. All of the skin and fat is lifted and pulled up toward the rib cage away from the abdomen. A hole is made around the belly button to leave it in position. Muscles which have become loosened are pulled together and stitched like an internal corset. These muscles now sit together as they had in the pre-pregnancy state. Skin and fat are pulled tightly down toward the pubic area creating a flatter look. Excess skin and fat are then excised. A new belly button opening is created in the repositioned skin. Liposuction is performed on the sides of the abdomen to feather and smooth the area. Two drains are placed, one on each side, which are inserted through another incision. These drains serve to remove fluids which accumulate during the surgery. Output from these drains is recorded to check fluid production, color, and amount of drainage. Patients undergoing a tummy tuck may have to remain in the hospital overnight. This overnight stay will usually be an additional expense of $ 750 -1000. Some patients return home or go to a hotel with a private duty nurse. In either scenario, someone must be available to assist you. Since there is moderate discomfort associated with a tummy tuck, your surgeon will likely prescribe pain medication as well as antibiotics.

Day One: Post—Operative Recovery Period

When you awake in the recovery room, you will notice that you are not lying flat. You will be in a "beach chair position" with your legs bent at the knees and your back will be elevated. This position reduces tension on the suture line and helps to minimize pulling that occurs if you lie flat. You will also notice two drains and possibly an abdominal binder which supports the skin and muscles and holds them in place. The drains will stay in anywhere from 3 days to 2 weeks and are an important part of the post-operative recovery. The abdominal compression garment will have to be worn for six weeks after surgery. On the third week, your surgeon will allow you to wear the garment only at night. Since you were given general anesthesia, your throat may be scratchy and dry.

Day One

The pain associated with a tummy tuck is typically less than that of a caesarean section, but worse than many other cosmetic procedures. On day one, you or your private duty nurse must empty the drains as per the instructions from your surgeon. You will record the amount of drainage as well as the color. You can expect about 40-80 cc per day of fluid with a reddish-whitish in color. These drains remove fluids that would cause swelling if allowed to accumulate. The removal of this fluid allows the skin to lie flat against the muscle.

You will notice that an incision scar is visible from hip to hip. Although the scar will look unsightly for the first few weeks, this will eventually fade over the course of several months.

Week One

If you have stayed in the hospital overnight, getting home may be difficult. You will likely experience some pain when you walk and may not be able to stand erect. You should sleep elevated with pillows behind your head and under your knees. If you have children at home, you may want to recruit some assistance to help care for them for a few days. You can anticipate swelling and bruising to increase over the next three days and will finally begin to plateau on day four. For the first three days, you may feel that the surgery was a mistake; that you never should have done it. These feelings are common and usually turnaround at day four or five when you are feeling much better. Cosmetic surgery typically creates an emotional rollercoaster and since tummy tuck surgery is more painful with a longer recovery than some others, the emotional peaks and valleys may be intensified. Do not become disappointed or concerned when you realize that you still cannot stand erect during the first week.

On day four or five, your surgeon will check your drains and incisions. The bandages are usually changed as well. It is a good idea to take some pain medication right before this post-op visit to reduce any discomfort associated with removal of your drains. The surgeon will be checking for any redness or inflammation and look for signs of healing in the navel area. One or both drains may be removed during this visit. Once this is done, you will begin to feel more comfortable. As you begin to feel better, you will think that this surgery wasn't such a bad idea after all! You can shower the day after your stitches or staples are removed. Use a gentle soap and warm water and let it fall gently over your skin and incisions. The steri-strips that help hold skin together will probably fall off during the first week. Do not pull them off; as they become loosened, they may be removed and replaced with new strips for six weeks. Approximately 5% of people have an allergic reaction to the steri-strips. If you see a red rash and inflammation, this may be an indication of such a reaction. Your surgeon will likely advise you to remove all of the steri-strips and apply moisturizer or topical antibiotic cream three times per day. You will still have significant swelling, especially in the areas in which liposuction was performed.

Weeks Two to Six

In week two or three, you should be able to return to work, but you may continue to have some discomfort. If you have had a prior caesarean section, you will notice that the recovery period is similar. At week six, you feel much better and can resume all of your normal activities.

At about six weeks, your new and flatter tummy will now be more apparent. Much of the swelling and bruising will have subsided. Fullness on the sides where liposuction incisions were made may still be visible and palpable for the first year. You will be returning to your surgeon for regular check-ups so that he or she can monitor your healing process.

It will take several weeks for the swelling to finally disappear so you should not be alarmed. As you look at your scars, you will notice them prominently for several weeks or months, but they will fade over time. In lighter-skinned people, a light scar line may still be visible even after a few years. Darker skinned individuals have more visible scarring and occasionally have scar hypertrophy in the first 9-12 months. If the scar becomes bumpy and does not fade or flatten out, your surgeon may have to perform a minor scar revision.

Pain Management

Since the tummy tuck is the most uncomfortable of all the procedures that we will be discussing, we thought it would be prudent to have a section devoted to pain management. The pain will vary depending on the type of tummy tuck performed. If the procedure involved tightening of muscles in addition to the excision of skin and fat, you can expect more discomfort. When your surgeon describes to you which procedure will be performed, you can get a general sense of the pain you can expect. Some patients experience a high variation of pain depending on their tolerance level, their compliance with medications and the procedure performed.

The good news is that there are new pain management devices which can effectively control pain in tummy tucks. A local anesthetic agent, Marcaine, is delivered under the skin through a tube which has been inserted. This tube delivers fluid and medication into the affected area, and essentially bathes the area with local anesthesia. This process works well in the first 2 or 3 days to control pain. Ask about this new Marcaine reservoir when you discuss your procedure with your surgeon.

Patients are usually sent home on oral pain medication as well. Take your medication as directed for at least three days to reduce discomfort. Remember that this is not the time to be a martyr or heroine. Increased levels of pain will increase blood pressure which can interfere with the healing process and cause complications. It is better all around if you reduce your discomfort and try to relax for the first several days after surgery. Healing is a delicate process which can be disturbed by excess activity.

The Mini-Tummy Tuck

This procedure removes skin and fatty tissue only below the belly button. There is less scarring and minimal surgery, but less improvement. This procedure is done when a patient has excess skin, but their muscles are not stretched out. Recovery time for the mini-tummy tuck is two weeks.

Significant Weight Loss

Obese patients who have undergone bariatric (obesity) surgery such as gastric by-pass or lap banding and have lost a significant amount of weight often seek body contouring. These patients have gone through extensive and complicated prior surgeries and have had significant changes in their weight, lifestyle, and metabolism. In some of these patients, it becomes a medical necessity to remove the unsightly excess skin and tissue which lies flaccid on their body. If not removed, this hanging tissue can become infected and irritated. These patients have physiologic, emotional, and anatomic nuances which must be assessed and treated in an individualized manner prior to surgery.

The complication rate for such things such as hematoma and poor wound healing in these patients is higher than for the average patient. There is a delicate balance between achieving the best cosmetic result while optimizing the safest post-operative course. Although many of the techniques are similar to a tummy tuck, the skin and blood vessels in these patients behave differently. The patients must be aware that the complication rates are higher for them and the healing process may be prolonged and require additional care. While the scarring may be more extensive, these patients are usually very satisfied with their result.

Many patients often explore contouring procedures soon after their bariatric procedure because they are thrilled with their weight loss and are ready to take the next step. They are advised, however, that they must be at their stable weight, which usually requires a year after their bariatric surgery before they can be considered for body contouring.

Unlike many cosmetic procedures, a tummy tuck or other tightening procedure performed after bariatric surgery may be covered by insurance. This will depend on your insurance coverage and reason for the surgery. If this sagging skin is creating discomfort or prolonged irritation or infection, some carriers will pay for the surgery. If financing is an issue, please confer with your insurance carrier prior to the procedure.

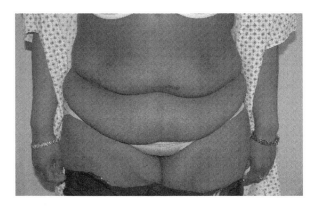

Tummy tuck front pre-op

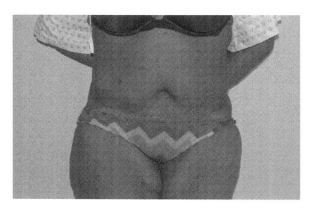

Tummy tuck front post-op

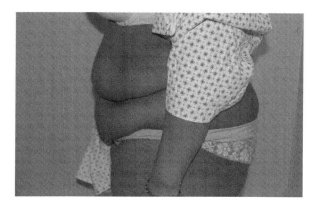

Tummy tuck side pre-op

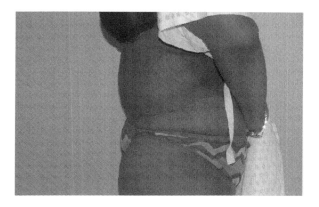

Tummy tuck side post-op

Do's and Don'ts

- Don't shower or bathe while the drains are in place
- Do shower 24 hours after the drains are removed
- Don't stretch or lie prone for the first few days after surgery
- Don't do aerobics for at least two weeks after surgery
- Don't consider a tummy tuck if you are planning to become pregnant in the near future
- Do keep pillows under the knees and sleep with your head elevated, or sleep on a recliner
- Don't panic if your tummy does not look flat immediately since there will be significant swelling which masks your new shape

Possible Complications

Listed below are some possible complications that may occur with this procedure. Your surgeon will review the possible complications with you when you are asked to consent for surgery.

- **Seroma:** This minor complication makes the abdomen appear fuller. You may require a minor in—office procedure to drain the fluid from the abdomen.
- **Bleeding:** It is possible, though unusual, to experience a bleeding episode during or after surgery. Should post-operative bleeding occur, it may require emergency treatment to drain accumulated blood or blood transfusion.
- **Infection:** Should an infection occur, treatment including antibiotics or additional surgery may be necessary.
- **Change in skin sensation and contour:** Diminished or loss of skin sensation in the lower abdominal area may not totally resolve after abdominoplasty. Contour irregularities such as wrinkling and depressions of the skin may also occur after abdominoplasty.
- **Delayed healing:** Some areas of the abdomen may not heal normally. This may require further wound care or additional surgery.
- **Pulmonary complications:** Pulmonary complications may occur because of blood clots (pulmonary emboli) after general anesthesia. You may require hospitalization and additional treatment. Pulmonary emboli can be life-threatening in some circumstances.
- **Umbilicus:** The belly button (navel) may not heal properly, scar, or necrose (die) following surgery.

CHAPTER 10
Eyelid Surgery (Blepharoplasty)

Pain scale: 3 out of 10
Procedure length: 1 hour for upper lids; 1 hour for lower lids
Return to Work Time: One week

The eyes are the main focal point when looking at someone's face. People are often evaluated by the look of their eyes. Terms like "Bright eyes" and "Ol' blue eyes" reflect the impact that the eyes have on the overall appearance. If your eyes are hidden by droopy skin, wrinkles, or fat deposits, it creates a tired, aged appearance that detracts from your looks. The biggest bang for your buck is eyelid surgery. This procedure is very popular because it yields the greatest improvement with the least recovery time or discomfort.

Indications for this surgery are upper eyelids that droop or sag over the eye, sometimes touching the eyelashes. There may also be puffiness in the inner corner of the eye or below the eye, which is caused by excess deposits of fat. Lower lids may sometimes look puffy resulting in a tired appearance. Sometimes the eyebrows look droopy, which can be corrected with a brow lift. Typical age of patients seeking eyelid surgery ranges from early 40s to 70s. Some patients are younger than 40 if they have a hereditary component which prematurely ages their eyelids. Most patients seeking eyelid surgery usually undergo upper and lower blepharoplasties at the same time. In some cases, however, only the upper or lower is needed, and only one procedure is performed. Blepharoplasty surgery will rejuvenate the eyes and improve the contour of the lid, creating a more awake and energetic look.

A Blepharoplasty will correct the following problems:
• Baggy upper eyelids (excess skin)
• Droopy upper eyelids

- Puffy upper eyelids (fat deposits)
- Puffy areas under the eyes
- Loose lower eyelids

A Blepharoplasty will not correct the following problems:

- Discoloration under the eyes
- Crow's feet (wrinkles on the sides of the eyes)
- Droopy eyebrows
- Droopy forehead
- Vision problems

Pre-Operative Considerations

If you have any eye problems such as dry eye, visual problems, or prior retinal detachments, you should discuss this with your surgeon prior to your surgery. Your surgeon may elect to send you to an ophthalmologist for an evaluation. If your eyes are puffy or swollen related to a thyroid disorder, you will need to see your endocrinologist for medical clearance prior to surgery.

Procedure

A Blepharoplasty is performed under light sedation and does not require an overnight stay. In a standing, upright position, your normal creases will be marked while you are in the holding area prior to surgery. Once you are sedated, local anesthesia is injected to your eyelid to further numb the area. The extra skin from your upper eyelids is removed and any excess fat from the middle or inner corner will be sculpted. For upper lids, the skin is usually closed with most of the sutures placed under the skin to prevent any visible scarring. The ends of the sutures are held in place by tape and can be removed easily later on.

For lower lids, the incisions are placed either inside the eyelid or outside the eyelid underneath the eyelashes. If there is excess fat to be removed, but no excess skin, the incision can be placed inside the eyelid. This technique is known as transconjunctival approach. The disadvantage of the inside incision is that excess skin under the eye cannot be excised. The advantage of this approach is that there is no visible scarring. If there is excess skin and excess fat, an incision below the eyelash is made and the excess skin is cut away. The lower incision will heal very nicely over the next few months. Once the excess skin and fat are excised, the skin is closed with very fine sutures. Sutures are usually removed on day three or four in your surgeon's office. Since there may be with some discomfort when removing these sutures, it is recommended that you take some Tylenol or pain medication before this visit to relieve any discomfort.

Day One: Post-Operative Recovery Period

You will wake up in the recovery room and there will be cool compresses on the eyes. When you open your eyes, your vision will be blurry. Do not be alarmed as this is completely normal and expected. Your surgeon applied some ointment in your eye for lubrication which causes the vision to become cloudy. This cloudiness will dissipate over the next few hours. You should keep your head elevated to minimize swelling, and cool compresses should be applied. You should expect some burning and itching at the suture line. Your surgeon will have prescribed pain medication for you when you go home. You will probably not have pain when you awaken in the recovery area because the local anesthesia has not yet worn off.

For the first night, keep lights low in your bedroom. Apply compresses every 15 minutes for the next 48 hours and keep your head elevated to minimize the swelling. Some patients feel more comfortable resting in a recliner; others prefer lying down with several pillows. You may notice some blood-tinged fluid draining from the sides of the eyes; this is normal. You will likely feel well enough to get up and be active on this first night, but you must force yourself to lie down, take your pain medication, and relax. Excessive activity will cause an increase in blood pressure and swelling which can lead to a collection of blood called a hematoma. If one eye is markedly more swollen than the other, or has increasing pain or pressure, or visual changes, call your surgeon immediately. These could be signs of a hematoma; this needs to be treated immediately.

Days Two to Three

As the days progress, you will notice more bruising and swelling which may not be equal on both sides. Eyes will be puffy, and you will not look pretty, much like someone who just lost a fight. In most cases, sutures will be removed in your surgeon's office on day three. The morning that you go to your surgeon for suture removal, take some pain medication to reduce discomfort. Your surgeon probably prescribed some ophthalmic ointment that should be applied to the suture lines. This will allow the sutures to be lubricated and allow them to slide out effortlessly with minimal discomfort. Once the sutures are removed, you will start to notice marked improvement. The swelling will subside and you will start to look better and better. Even with some bruising and discoloration, you will see a more youthful appearance emerging.

Weeks One To Six

Over the next week, your bruising will subside and the contour and shape will improve. Cover-up makeup can be used to camouflage bruising and allow you to return to work and normal activity. Over the next two to six weeks, the bruising will dissipate and the coloration will lighten. The scars will heal over the next several months and be very difficult to find after a year. In two to six weeks, you may feel a small pimple on the outer edge of your lower eyelid—this is from a stitch placed under the skin to hold everything in place. This stitch usually dissolves in six weeks. If it does not dissolve, the surgeon may easily remove the stitch in his office. The procedure is no more complicated than removing a splinter.

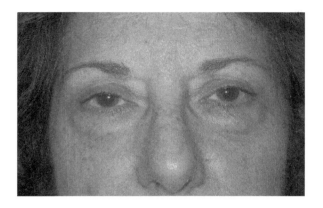

Blepharoplasty pre-op

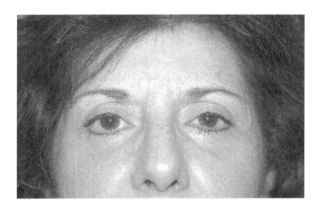

Blepharoplasty post-op

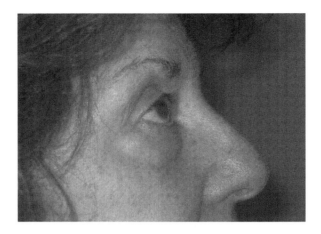

Blepharoplasty side pre-op

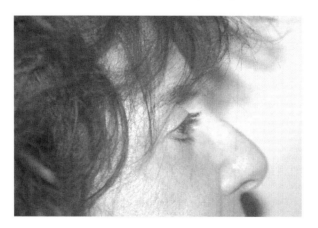

Blepharoplasty side post-op

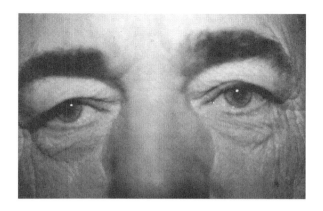

Blepharoplasty pre-op

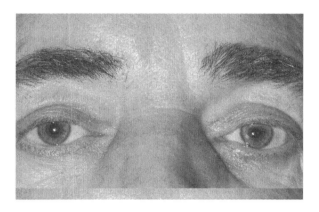

Blepharoplasty, post-op

Do's and Don'ts

- Do help promote healing. At the health food store, you can find Arnica cream which can be applied on the surface of the cheeks to help reduce the bruising and swelling
- Do apply cover-up make up to the bruised area 24 hours after sutures are removed if so desired
- Do purchase artificial tears over the counter in any pharmacy if your eyes are dry
- Don't pull the eyelids or eyebrows or rub your eyes if they itch. Glasses may be worn as needed

- Don't wear contacts until cleared by your surgeon. This may require two to six weeks depending on your surgery
- Don't apply any eye make up such as mascara for two days after sutures have been removed
- Do see your surgeon if you notice some white pimples, known as milia on the suture lines; these can be easily cleaned in the office

Possible Complications

Listed below are some possible complications that may occur with this procedure. Your surgeon will review the possible complications with you when you are asked to consent for surgery.

- **Bleeding:** Significant bleeding after blepharoplasty is rare. Some dripping of blood from the eye onto your skin is not an emergency. Any minor bleeding will usually stop on its own. If, on the other hand, one eye becomes hardened, swollen, or significantly more painful than the other eye, this is a sign of internal bleeding (hematoma). Hematomas require immediate attention; however, the treatment is quite simple. Often with the removal of one stitch, the hematoma can be relieved. Sometimes, further medical or surgical treatment is required.
- **Blindness:** Exceedingly rare, blindness has been reported with blepharoplasty, due to the pressure of a hematoma.
- **Damage to deeper structures:** Eye muscles could be damaged during this procedure that could result in double vision. This may be temporary or require additional surgery.
- **Dry eye and corneal exposure:** After blepharoplasty surgery, your eyes may be dry and irritated. Individuals who normally have dry eyes are at greater risk of having this complication. Some patients have difficulty closing their eyelids after surgery and problems may occur in the cornea due to dryness. Should this rare complication occur, additional treatments or surgery and treatment may be necessary.
- **Ectropion:** Displacement of the lower eyelid away from the eyeball is a rare complication. Further surgery may be required to correct this condition.

CHAPTER 11
Brow lift

Pain scale: 6 out of 10
Length of Procedure: 1.5—2 hours
Return to Work Time: 1—2 weeks

The Brow lift smoothes lines between the eyebrows or on the forehead and creates a youthful arched shape to the eyebrows. A brow lift is best suited for those people whose eyebrows have changed positions or are drooping. Depending on where they are drooping, and the appearance of the forehead, there are several procedures for brow lifts. The most common area for droopiness is toward the outside of the eye. This sagging creates heaviness of the upper lid causing it to hang over the eyelashes. If the brow is pulled up and arched over the side of the eye, it can immediately improve your image. The trick to this procedure is to regulate the amount of lift. If the brow is lifted too much, a startled or "deer in the headlights" look is created. For a more natural look, it is imperative that the surgeon be skilled at this procedure. You do not want a dramatic change from a brow lift, only a slight improvement, creating a youthful appearance.

Brow lifts are often done in concert with an upper blepharoplasty, but they be performed as a single procedure, too. There are several different techniques that can be used for a Brow lift, each with its own set of advantages and disadvantages.

A Brow lift is an ambulatory procedure with sedation anesthesia. You are able to go home approximately one hour after the procedure has been completed. There are three basic types of brow list procedures: The Coronal approach, the Endoscopic technique, and the Subcutaneous approach.

Coronal lift

The standard procedure for brow lifting is the coronal lift which extends from ear to ear across the scalp. The scalp is incised and pulled backwards away from the forehead. The advantage is that you can get a significant lift that is long lasting and eliminates wrinkling in the forehead. The disadvantage is that it is a more invasive approach, which may result in hair loss and numbness. A less invasive, modified version of the Coronal lift is sometimes used, which lifts the lateral part of the eyebrow only and does not cause as much sensory loss.

Endoscopic lift

The Endoscopic technique is a newer technique introduced in the early 1990s. This procedure is less invasive than the older Coronal lift. In this procedure, small incisions are used at specified areas in the scalp where tiny endoscopes are inserted under the skin and scalp. Endoscopes allow the surgeon to view nerves and muscles under the scalp without the need to cut it completely open. The endoscope is a mini-telescope with a camera that allows the surgeon to view the delicate anatomy magnified on a television monitor. These enhancements allow for more precise and safer surgery. The surgeon can directly view the nerves that supply sensation to the forehead and scalp and keep them in tact to avoid numbness or permanent loss of sensation. The forehead is then lifted up and secured into a new position. When this procedure first became available, many surgeons embraced it because of all these benefits. Although the advantages of this procedure are significant, over time, some surgeons have noted that the results are not as long lasting as the traditional Coronal approach.

An excellent option for many brow lifts is a modified Endoscopic approach with both incisions on the sides as well as tiny incisions in the middle of the scalp. The marriage of these two techniques allows the surgeon to maximize the benefits of both while minimizing the disadvantages. This modified technique utilizes larger incisions on the sides that contribute to longer lasting results, combined with smaller incisions in the middle of the scalp, which facilitate the endoscopic visualization.

Subcutaneous lift

The Subcutaneous lift is a procedure where only the upper layer of skin is pulled back with an incision in front of the hairline. This is used for patients with high foreheads because it will not increase the length of the forehead when the skin is lifted and tightened. A disadvantage of this technique is a visible scar at the hairline.

Your surgeon will review different options with you and choose the best procedure for you depending on your anatomy and desired outcome.

Post-operative course

You will awaken in the recovery room and notice that your upper eyelids are swollen and you may have a headache at the top of the head. Over the next two to three days, the swelling progresses and the forehead and eyes will feel swollen. Some bruising will be noticed on the cheeks. You may receive some steroid medication to reduce the swelling. You may be uncomfortable because of the swelling, but will probably not experience sharp or shooting pain. Your surgeon will prescribe pain medication which you can take for the first two or three days. After that period, you will likely be able to control any discomfort with extra strength Tylenol.

To close the incisions, some surgeons use screws while others use sutures. In either case, closures are removed in two weeks. Screws may cause tiny protrusions in your scalp which may cause alarm. These protrusions are painless, uneventful, and will disappear when the screws are removed. Your hair may be thinning at the incision sites but these areas are hidden and this will be temporary as the hair grows back. Apply cool compresses for two days to reduce swelling. In six weeks, all of the swelling will be gone and you will see the new shape of your brow and forehead.

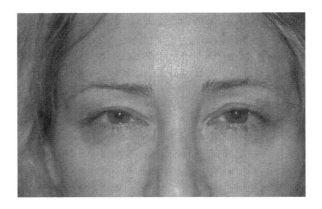

Brow lift pre-op

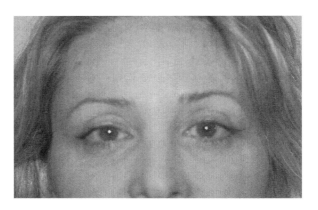

Brow lift post-op

Possible Complications

Listed below are some possible complications that may occur with this procedure. Your surgeon will review the possible complications with you when you are asked to consent for surgery.

- **Skin scarring and hair loss:** Wherever incisions are made, there may be scarring or hair loss
- **Nerve injury:** There is the potential for injury to both motor and sensory nerves during a brow lift procedure. This nerve injury may cause a temporary lack of motion or sensation in a portion of the forehead. After several months, the sensation and movement should return to normal. Weakness or loss in

movements of the forehead or upper eyebrow may occur after surgery

- **Hair loss:** Hair loss is a risk of this procedure because there are incisions made in the scalp. After several months, the hair will usually grow back although in rare cases, the loss may be permanent. This risk can be minimized by certain techniques
- **Hardware:** Some techniques require the use of screws or holes drilled in to the skull which can represent a risk of intracranial injury

CHAPTER 12
Ear Pinning (Otoplasty)

Pain scale: 5 out of 10
Procedure Time: 2—3 hours
Return to Work or School Time: 1—2 weeks

This procedure is commonly performed on children who were born with ears that protrude from their scalp. In addition to protruding, they are often missing some of the contours that constitute the shape of a normal ear. An Otoplasty is a procedure in which the ears are reshaped and pulled closer to the scalp.

When should your child have this surgery? For several reasons, this surgery should be performed at the age of five or six. Children between the ages of one and five tend to play independently and do not interact significantly. At the age of five or six, children have more interactive play and begin to notice and point out each others' faults. Teasing and name-calling become common in this age group. A five year old child with protruding ears is an easy target for other children to ridicule and tease. Some children can become emotionally distraught because of their physical imperfections. By age five, a child's ear has attained 80% of its adult size and is an appropriate time for surgical correction. Also by age five or six, children may be more tolerant and compliant with the procedure.

This procedure is not limited to children. Many adults, who, for whatever reason did not have surgery as a child, seek intervention later in life. These adults may have been ridiculed all through school and throughout their adolescent life.

Procedure

In adults, the procedure is performed under MAC anesthesia. A small amount of sedation is used with local anesthesia administered around the ears. Children, however, are frightened, and are placed under general anesthesia. This is the safest option for children and allows the surgeon to get the best results.

An incision is made behind the ear to gain access to the cartilage. From this hidden incision area, all of the sculpting is performed. In this technique, the most natural result is achieved, but there is a chance that the sutures can loosen, which result in loss of the new contouring. An alternative technique can be performed, which results in a more permanent result, but it are not nearly as natural looking in appearance. There are typically two main objectives of this procedure. The first is to remove the excess cartilage that is pushing the ear away from the scalp. The ear can then be repositioned closer to the head. The second objective is to reshape the remaining cartilage into a normal appearing ear. This reshaping is often done with sutures, which remain under the skin. This is important to understand for the post operative course. The surgeon will finish one ear, and using measurements, tries to recreate the closest possible match so that the ears look as similar as possible. The skin incision is closed with the excess skin being removed.

Recovery Period

When you awaken, you will notice that there is gauze wrapping around the head and ears. The local anesthetic will still be active, so the areas will still be numb. Sounds will be muffled due to the bandages on the ears. Approximately three hours later, the local anesthetic wears off and you will feel some mild throbbing involving both ears. Your dressing may get slightly stained with blood. This is done purposely because the closure is not water tight, allowing the blood to drip out. You should take your pain medication and antibiotics as prescribed. You should sleep with your head elevated with two pillows behind your head.

Day One

You will return to see your surgeon the following day and your dressing will be changed. Your surgeon is checking to see that no blood has collected under the skin, forming a hematoma. If he does find this collection, he may aspirate it with a needle or remove a stitch to drain it. This is done to insure that the skin heals well and produces the best cosmetic result. You may start to shower twenty four hours after surgery. You may apply antibiotic ointment behind the ears on the incision, and your surgeon will probably give you a headband to wear to keep the ears in their new position. It is important for the first three weeks to wear this band as much as possible, especially when you sleep, to avoid the ear bending forward.

Weeks One to Three

For the first two weeks, the ears will be swollen and itchy. At week three to six, the swelling dissipates significantly and the final new shape is noticeable. Small incremental changes will continue to occur over the next few weeks and months. You may feel a tiny hairlike, splintery protrusion behind the ear. This suture can easily be removed in the office.

Returning to Work and School

A child can return to school one to two weeks after surgery. The ears are delicate for the first two weeks and need to be protected. The child has to avoid physical contact sports for six weeks to prevent damage to the ear. After six weeks, all physical activities can be resumed. An adult can return to work one week later, but should avoid any strenuous physical activity.

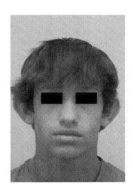

Otoplasty pre-op

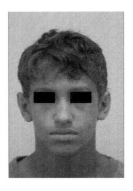

Otoplasty post-op

(Photos courtesy of Samuel M. Lam, M.D.)

Do's and Don'ts
- Do wear the headband as prescribed by your physician
- Don't wear any protective helmets
- Do advise your surgeon of any increased pain, redness, or swelling
- Do refrain from sports for six weeks

Possible Complications
Listed below are some possible complications that may occur with this procedure. Your surgeon will review the possible complications with you when you are asked to consent for surgery.

- **Hematoma:** Swelling in the surgical site may develop into a collection of blood called a hematoma. If there is marked pain or swelling in one ear over the other, you should notify your physician immediately
- **Infection:** Infection can occur after Otoplasty. There can be increased redness, swelling, or pain in one or both ears. It is especially important in Otoplasty to take your antibiotics. If any of these signs appear, please call your physician
- **Ear trauma:** Ears are sensitive for the first six weeks after surgery. Accidental trauma to the ear may distort the results of the surgery
- **Asymmetry:** As with all cosmetic surgical procedures, there

may be some asymmetry following surgery. This may be due to scarring, healing or pre-operative asymmetry

- **Recurrence:** It is possible that the stitches in the cartilage may not hold the ear shape in place and the shape may revert back to normal. This may require revision surgery

CHAPTER 13
Breast Augmentation

Pain scale: 8 out of 10
Procedure time: 1- 2 hours
Return to Work Time: 2 weeks

B reast augmentation is the third most common procedure with more than 350,000 procedures performed in 2006. The typical patients seeking breast augmentation are women in their 30s and 40s, although the trend has been toward younger women. This procedure involves an extensive consultation with your surgeon.

Choice of Implant:
There are several variables in breast augmentations.
- The choice of implant
- The incision to gain access to place the implant
- The location of the implant

There are several varieties of implants. They can be smooth or textured (like stucco) and can be round or naturally shaped like a tear drop. Different surgeons have different preferences depending on the breast shape of the patient. The round implant is more commonly used by surgeons because, if it moves around, it still retains its shape. The round shape also provides more cleavage to the patient. When a patient stands up, the round shape forms a tear drop due to gravity. Some surgeons prefer the teardrop because it resembles a natural breast shape; but, if the teardrop rotates by accident, the shape will be distorted.

The most important part of breast augmentation is picking the right size. This is the most common thing that patients wish they could do over. Take your time when thinking about this. This is not the time to by shy with your physician. There are several ways that your physician can determine the right size for you. He will give you several sizes of actual implants that you can place inside your bra. You can place a shirt over it the implant and get a ballpark idea of what you may look like after the procedure. Note, these implants will not correlate exactly with the size that you need. You will get a "feel" of the sizes and what makes you comfortable.

The next trick, which may sound silly, is to go home and fill zip lock bags with different amounts of rice. Place the different sizes into your bra until your find the size that looks good to you. When you find the right size, bring it to your surgeon. He will correlate this size with the typical implant sizes which range from 200-600 ccs. Another option is to buy an inexpensive bra that is your desired size. Fill this bra with these bags of rice and bring the bag to your physician. The physician will measure the volume. In addition to these results, the surgeon will assess your height and weight, dimension of your chest and body shape. He will consider all of these variables to determine the right size of implant. As you can see, the sizing is more complicated than you may have thought and needs to be a joint decision between you and your surgeon.

The Procedure

There are several options for placing the implant. Each surgeon has his preference and there are advantages and disadvantages to each one. The standard approaches for insertion include around the aureola, under the breast, through the armpit, and through the navel.

This procedure is usually performed under general anesthesia, with local anesthesia added to the breast site to decrease discomfort when you wake up. The procedure takes approximately 90-120 minutes. You will be able to go home the same day of the procedure.

There are several techniques used for breast augmentation:

Under the breast: A 2-inch incision is made on each side and a pocket is made under the breast tissue or under the chest muscle. The implant is placed inside and filled with the appropriate amount of salt water. The incision is closed using a plastic surgery technique. Over several months, this incision heals nicely and, unless someone looks underneath, the scar is invisible. Patients are generally very satisfied with this procedure. The advantage of this technique is that it is easier for the surgeon to create a pocket for the implant and control bleeding. The disadvantage, albeit small, is the scar on the underside of the breast.

Peri-aureolar (around the nipple): The incision here is made on the bottom half of the nipple; this is where access is gained to place the implant. This is suitable for women with larger aureola. Some surgeons feel that this heals very nicely, but there is a higher chance of sensory changes to the nipple

Armpit placement: A 2 inch incision is placed in the armpit. Specialized pieces of equipment such as endoscopes are used to create the pocket in the breast and place the implant. This placement is not recommended for taller women because it is technically complex. The distance from the armpit to the bottom of the implant is far which makes the procedure difficult. In shorter women who do not mind a scar, it may be a good choice. When wearing sleeveless garments, the scar from this procedure may be visible. The benefit is that there is no scar on the breast.

Navel placement: The Incision is placed inside the navel and specialized equipment is used to create a pocket and place the implant. The advantage is that there is no scar on the breast. The disadvantage is that it is harder for the surgeon to get the implant in perfect position and control bleeding.

The most important part is not which technique is used. Your surgeon will help guide you in the decision. It is more important for you to understand the implications of surgery and the long term effects of having implants.

In breast augmentation, the surgeon is inserting prosthesis into your body. Whenever a foreign material is introduced into the body, many complications may occur. You must be informed not only about the procedure, but what lifelong implications are involved. This surgery is different than others which primarily remove and reshape excess skin and fat. In a breast augmentation, a foreign body implant is inserted into the body. There is no guarantee how the body will react to this foreign body.

It is no secret that 12 years ago, the FDA banned silicone implants. Many have seen the talk shows and read articles about women who had serious illnesses, which they alleged were caused by their implants. Since that time, many scientific studies have been done. None of these studies found a medical link between silicone implants and auto-immune diseases. Currently, silicone implants can only be used in investigational studies while additional research on them is being conducted. Cosmetic procedures in this country commonly use saline (salt water) implants. Note that the outer shell is still made of the silicone material, but the inside is saline fluid rather than silicone through and through. When silicone implants were banned, volume of breast augmentations dropped significantly. Over the past 14 years, studies have demonstrated the safety of saline implants. Also, the concern of silicone causing auto-immune disorders has not been proven and some of the apprehension has dissipated. Over the past few years, the volume of these procedures is once again on the rise.

Recovery Period

When you wake up in the recovery room, you will be wearing a surgical bra, which helps to support the new breasts. At first, you will look down and touch them and worry that your new breasts are too large. Do not be alarmed; there is swelling after surgery. This swelling will take several weeks to subside. There will be little discomfort when you awaken in the recovery room because of the local anesthetic. By the time you get home, the local anesthetic will wear off and you will experience some discomfort. (When surgeons say discomfort, that usually means pain.) Ask your surgeon to provide these prescriptions before your surgery so that you can be prepared when you get home. Take the pain medication as prescribed by your surgeon.

Within the first 24 hours, you have to be on the lookout for several complications. Sudden enlargement of one breast could be an indication of a hematoma which is a collection of blood under the skin. This condition is extremely painful and may require a trip to the operating room for draining. If you suspect a hematoma, you should call your surgeon immediately.

The next morning, you will wake up and you may think that the procedure was not worth the discomfort. The pain medication will help reduce the pain, but you will likely be feeling some discomfort. As in some other procedures, you will likely ask yourself, "Why did I do this?" If the implant is placed under the muscle, it will likely be more painful than if the implant is placed under the skin. You will be given antibiotics and you will take as prescribed that first day after surgery. Taking these antibiotics is important because a foreign object has been inserted into your body. If this implant got infected, it would have to be removed. Taking the antibiotics may help with healing and prevent complications later on.

Week One

Over the next three days, your breasts will typically continue to swell. After the fourth day, the swelling starts to subside. One breast may initially feel softer or appear larger than the other. This is due to swelling around the implant and may occur unevenly. People may initially think that one breast is leaking or the implants are not the same size. After six weeks, the swelling will have resolved and both breasts will look more similar is size.

Any gauze that is under the bra may be changed as necessary. During this time, just wear the bra your doctor put on you in the operating room. You may typically shower after the second day, but do not remove any steri-strips over the incision sites. On your first post-operative appointment (within the first two weeks), your physician will change the steri-strips. By this point, you are beginning to like the shape and realize the benefits of the surgery. If you have a child, it is wise to line up a babysitter to help you. It may be difficult to lift for the first few days, so you should limit activities. If you have temperature or increased redness of the skin of the breast, warmth of the breast, or increased tenderness, you should call your surgeon since this may be the beginning of an infection.

Week Two
Within the first two weeks, your surgeon will remove the steri-strips. The sutures are usually dissolvable and do not need to be removed. In addition, at two weeks, your surgeon will teach you how to massage the breasts. This will prevent scarring and capsular contraction which is scar tissue which tightens up around the implant. In the first two weeks, this massage should be gentle and over time should get more vigorous to help the breast tissue around the implant remain soft and supple. For the first two weeks, there is no exercising allowed. After two weeks, lower body exercise is allowed. Full exercising is permitted only after six weeks.

Six Weeks
At this point, you will out in an evening dress and you will glance at your new figure. You will be comfortable with your new size and may even wish that you went bigger! Most patients forget by now that the procedure was uncomfortable and would do it again in a second.

It takes some time to adjust to your new shape. You should be made aware of new sensations. If you have a saline implant, it is common to hear a swishing sound for the first few weeks. It is also common to feel or see rippling of the skin on top of the implant. This is more noticeable in women with smaller breasts or thinner breast tissue. For this reason, the surgeon may choose to place the implant under the muscle. Some women have reported that the saline implant may create a cold sensation under the skin in very cold temperatures. Don't worry; these implants will not freeze in your body.

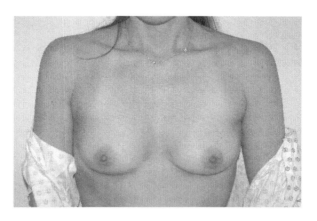

Breast Augmentation pre-op

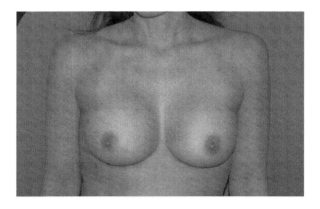

Breast Augmentation post-op

Do's and Don'ts
- Do notify your surgeon of increasing temperature, redness, or pain

- Don't be alarmed if you think they are too large; remember, there is increased swelling
- Do massage as prescribed by your surgeon to prevent capsular contraction
- Do wear the bra that was prescribed by your surgeon

Possible Complications

Listed below are some possible complications that may occur with this procedure. Your surgeon will review the possible complications with you when you are asked to consent for surgery.

- **Capsular contraction:** Scar tissue forms internally around the implant, which causes the breast to become firm and painful. This complication may occur weeks or months after the implants have been inserted. Despite excellent surgical technique, there is no way to predict who will get this complication. If this occurs, and the shape of the breast is unnatural, you may elect to have your implants replaced or removed entirely. This would require additional surgery.
- **Hematoma:** After the surgery, one breast may be more painful or markedly larger than the other. These are signs of a hematoma which is a collection of blood under the breast. If this occurs, you must notify your physician. Your physician may elect to perform additional surgery to evacuate the hematoma.
- **Infection:** Infection is not common after breast augmentation, but may occur immediately following the procedure or at any other time. You must keep in mind that the implant is a foreign body that may become infected sometime in the future. If you do develop an infection, antibiotic therapy, possible removal of the implant, or additional surgery may be necessary.
- **Change in nipple and skin sensation:** Some change in nipple sensation is not unusual right after surgery. After several months, most patients have normal sensation. Partial or permanent loss of nipple and skin sensation may occur occasionally as a result of this procedure.
- **Implant Damage:** When a woman seeks implants, it is important to understand that, unlike diamonds, implants

do not last forever. Implants can rupture or leak either from trauma, during mammography, or for no apparent reason. If an implant is damaged or has a leak, it will need to be replaced or removed, which will require additional surgery. Over the course of ten years, on average, half of the women will have their implants changed or removed.

- **Implant extrusion:** Skin and tissue breakdown due to injury or infection could result in exposure and/or extrusion of the implant. Removal of the implant may be necessary if this occurs.

- **Mammography:** Implant rupture can occur from during mammography. It is important that you inform your mammography technologist if you have breast implants before your exam. The appropriate mammogram studies must be obtained so that a proper screening can be performed. Patients with implants may experience more pain during a mammography if they have some capsular contraction. If a lump is detected, specialized mammography procedures and/or sonograms may be necessary for further evaluation.

- **Skin wrinkling and rippling:** Some wrinkling of the skin is normal and expected after augmentation. Patients who have saline implants or thin breast tissue may experience more rippling than they had expected. Each patient has different skin and tissue consistency, which may cause a slightly different appearance on the surface of the skin.

- **Pregnancy and breast feeding:** There is not sufficient scientific evidence to prove or refute whether there are increased safety risks for breast feeding or if the babies of women with breast implants are more likely to have health problems. Research is on-going in this arena and it is likely that some conclusions will be forthcoming in the future. If this is a major concern for you, please discuss in depth with your surgeon.

- **Implant migration:** Unanticipated movement of a breast implant may occur from its initial placement. This may result in pain, asymmetry, or distortion of the shape of the breast. You may require additional surgery to treat this problem.

CHAPTER 14
Breast Reduction

Pain Scale: 4 out of 10
Procedure time: 3 hours
Return to Work Time: 2 weeks

This procedure reduces the size of a woman's breasts and restores the natural lift of the breast. The ideal candidates are those women who have large breasts (such as size D or larger) and whose breasts are hanging or uncomfortable physically. There is no typical age range of women seeking this procedure. When the ideal candidate goes ahead with a reduction, they are usually extremely happy with the result. They feel like they can move around better, can exercise better, and feel better about themselves despite the visible scarring on the breasts. The patient should have a lengthy conversation with their surgeon to discuss the possibility of breast reduction and the extensive scarring. If you are a darker-skinned woman, the scar can become hypertropic or form keloids.

As part of a pre-operative physical, all patients having a breast reduction should have a mammogram to rule out any malignancies. Breast reduction is one of the few procedures which may be covered by insurance. If the surgery is being performed to resolve chronic back pain, neck pain, or bra strap grooving, you should have your internist forward letters to your plastic surgeon. Your surgeon can use this information along with his/her own note to request a pre-authorization to determine coverage from your insurance carrier.

The Procedure
Several techniques can be used for breast reduction. Most commonly, it involves making an incision around the aureola (nipple) down the middle of the breast and underneath in the crease area forming a T

shape. This allows your surgeon to excise part of the breast, remold it and lift the nipple to a higher position. Extra skin is cut away while the new breast is sculpted. The new breasts will be perkier, have a better shape, and be smaller in size. In very droopy breasts, sometimes the nipple is removed and regrafted in place. This technique may result in discoloration, scarring, or loss of nipple sensation. If your surgeon intends on performing this procedure, you should have a thorough discussion with him about these possible side effects.

Breast reduction is performed under general anesthesia. A drain is applied to each breast during the procedure. The drain allows the fluid and blood to flow out of the body and not accumulate under the skin.

Day One

You will awaken in the recovery room and may be nauseous from the anesthesia. Breast reduction surgery typically causes more nausea than other types of procedures. Your surgeon will order anti-nausea medication, which will be administered to you after the surgery to help you feel as comfortable as possible. You will feel tired after the general anesthesia and likely spend several hours in the recovery room. You will be wearing a special surgical bra which helps to support the new breast. You should only wear this bra or one that your surgeon recommends for six weeks. No underwire bras should be worn. You should not be concerned when you notice that drains have been placed; these are to remain for 24 hours.

You will look down and want to evaluate your new breasts. They will probably look larger than you were expecting because of swelling. You will go to your surgeon for a post-operative check-up on the first day after surgery. At this visit, the drains will be removed and you will be given pain medication and antibiotics. All medications should be taken as prescribed.

Week One

Your breasts, during this time period, will be numb and swollen. When you go home, you may expect that the gauze covering your incisions will be stained with blood. You should change this gauze as necessary, but do not shower. It is important that you do not get the breasts or the bandages across the suture lines wet. Sometime during the first week, you will see your physician for another post-operative check-up. At this visit, he will remove the steri-strips on the wounds and take out some of the sutures. Many of sutures are under the skin and will dissolve in the body. As these sutures dissolve, the swelling will dissipate. New steri-strips will be applied at this visit.

When you return home, you may resume showering. You will notice that the steri-strips may become loosened after several days. This is completely normal and should not be worrisome. At some point, some of the steri-strips will fall off. When this occurs, you should dry the incision line with a clean white towel and re-apply the steri-strips. This process is not essential, but if done for about six weeks from the date of surgery, will greatly benefit the healing process. The purpose of the steri-strips is to remove tension from the incision line and prevent the skin from pulling. This results in better healing and decreases the width of the scar. Your scars may be finer and smoother if you follow this easy procedure.

About ten percent of individuals have an allergic reaction to the steri-strips. You will notice that the skin under the strip becomes red and itchy. If this occurs, do not re-apply new steri-strips when the old ones fall off. In severe reactions, your surgeon will give you topical hydrocortisone or Benedryl to relieve the symptoms.

Two to Six Weeks

You should not be experiencing discomfort at this point. Although you may feel well enough to exercise, continue to refrain from heavy activity. For the first two weeks, sleep as much as possible on your back. After two weeks, you can start to sleep on your sides. At six weeks, it will not do any harm to sleep on your stomach, if that is your preferred manner of sleeping.

Two weeks after surgery, you may still be worried about the size of your new breasts. The swelling has started to subside but they still appear larger than you had expected. Over the next weeks and months, the size and shape will become more permanent. After two weeks, you can start stationery bicycling and lower body exercising.

Between two and six weeks, you will see the bruising and swelling continue to improve. You can slowly return to upper body activities. At six weeks you may go back to your regular bra and resume all physical activities. During this time period, it is not uncommon to see clear fluids seep out of the suture lines. Clear drainage with no pain associated is a normal part of the healing process. If, however, your breasts are red and tender, accompanied by pain and/or fever, you must notify your physician.

Scarring and Healing

Remember that the entire process of healing requires a full year. The shape will get smoother and rounder during this time period. The scars will continue to fade, but each patient's skin heals differently. This is not necessarily related to the surgeon or the procedure, but more on your own body's ability to heal. Dark-skinned individuals, such as African-Americans or Latinos, commonly have keloiding or hypertrophic scarring. If you have had problems with healing or scarring in the past, you should discuss this with your surgeon prior to the procedure. You will see your physician every four months during the first year. At these visits, your surgeon will examine the scars to see if they are healing well. If there is any keloiding or thickened scarring, there are several options for treatment.

- Topical silicone or steroid tapes can be applied, or scar fading ointments can be used
- Sometimes, your surgeon will elect to inject the steroid directly into the scar

Many patients over the course of a year are satisfied with the healing. After a year if the patient is not happy with the healing, the surgeon may elect to perform a minor scar revision procedure (see scar revision chapter for more information). After six weeks, you do not need to apply the steri-strips but you may apply topical Vitamin E three times a day to the scars. This may be done for up to a year to promote healing.

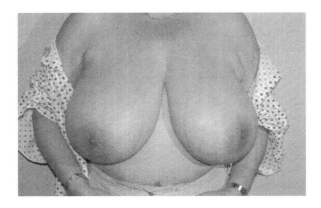

Breast Reduction pre-op

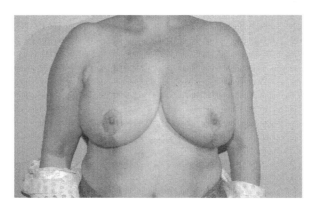

Breast Reduction post-op

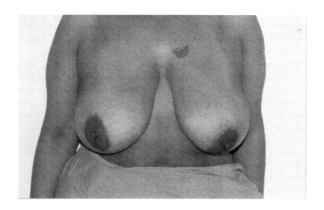

Breast Reduction pre-op

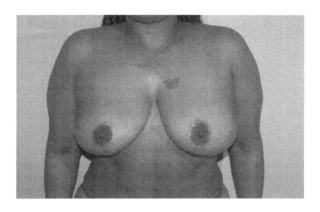

Breast Reduction post-op

Do's and Don'ts

- Do try to be at a stable weight. Drastic weight reduction after surgery may cause the breast to get even smaller.
- Do understand that there will be significant scarring on the breast that will be permanent but can be hidden by your bra.
- Do be patient and allow it to heal for a year.
- Don't go jogging for the first six weeks
- Don't sleep on your stomach for the first six weeks
- Don't pull off the steri-strips until they begin to peel off

Possible Complications

Listed below are some possible complications that may occur with this procedure. Your surgeon will review the possible complications with you when you are asked to consent for surgery

- **Infection**: Usually exhibited by increased redness, tenderness and fever. Sometimes, there may be a foul smelling fluid seeping from the incision sites. Infection can occur any time within the first four weeks. Your physician will want to see you and will prescribe a course of antibiotics.
- **Skin necrosis**: Although this is rare, a part of the wound sometimes may not heal well and may appear dark colored and scabby. You may be asked to apply topical antibiotic ointment such as Neosporin or Bacitracin. This complication occurs most commonly in patients who are smokers. Make sure you stop smoking for two weeks prior to surgery.
- **Loss of nipple sensation**: This can happen immediately after surgery and is a known risk of this procedure. Normal sensation may not occur for up to 18 months after the surgery.

CHAPTER 15
Breast Lift (Mastopexy)

Pain scale: 2 out of 10
Length of Procedure: 2 hours
Return to Work time: I week

A breast lift is similar in many ways to a breast reduction except that unlike a reduction that makes the cup size smaller, a lift does not reduce the size of the breast; it simply tightens the skin and lifts the existing breast upward. Ptotic (the medical term for droopy) or droopy breasts are not uncommon in many women. This droopiness occurs after weight loss, pregnancy, and breast feeding. Because of age, gravity, and pregnancy, many women's' breasts become ptotic. Larger breast have a tendency to hang more. Some women, although happy with their cup size, want to improve the shape of the breast. This procedure will help to reduce drooping and sagginess and result in a more youthful appearance.

The Procedure
There are several choices for a breast lift. One approach will leaves the least visible scarring is to place a small implant under the breast. This procedure is for someone who wants to increase the size and lift the breast. If a woman does not desire larger breasts, for a small lift, incisions are made around the aureola, skin is excised, and the nipple is lifted to a new position. For larger lifts, more incisions are required around the aureola, and down the breast iand sometimes in the infra-mammary crease. Basically, the greater the lift required, the more scarring you can expect. In larger lifts, you can have scarring similar to that of a breast reduction. A T-shaped incision is made, excess skin is removed, and the new breast shape is placed higher on the chest and sutured using plastics surgery technique. This procedure is done under general anesthesia and does not require any drains. Steri-strips are applied over the scars and a special surgical bra is worn after the surgery.

Recovery Period

You may have nausea when you awaken from this procedure as it is a common side effect in breast procedures. You will likely not experience much discomfort from this type of surgery. Your surgeon will prescribe pain medication and antibiotics for you to take over the next several days. You will have to wear a surgical bra for the next three weeks. There will be some bruising and swelling, which will dissipate over the next six weeks. You will visit your surgeon one week after surgery and your stitches will be removed. Do not shower until after your first visit with your surgeon.

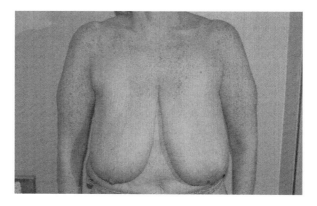

Breast Lift, front pre-op

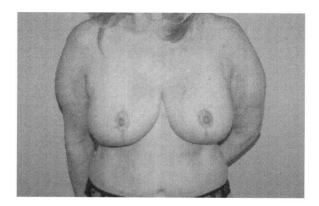

Breast Lift, front post-op

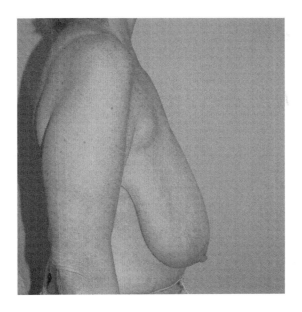

Breast Lift, side pre-op

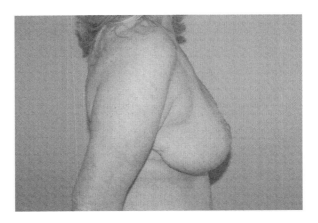

Breast Lift, side post-op

Possible Complications

Listed below are some possible complications that may occur with this procedure. Your surgeon will review the possible complications with you when you are asked to consent for surgery.

- **Bleeding**: Rapid enlargement or swelling of one breast greater than the other. This can be treated by draining the fluid. Sometimes, there may be a necessity to undergo another procedure to control the e bleeding.
- **Symmetry and Scarring**: There may be irregular scarring with poor healing. The scars are visible in a breast lift. There will always be a permanent scar, but it should hopefully improve over time. If the scars become thickened and raised, silicone sheeting may be applied over the scars in an effort to improve them. Despite accurate measuring, it could also heal asymmetrically. As with all cosmetic procedures, you may require additional corrective surgery.
- **Loss of nipple sensation**: This is always a risk of breast surgery. Sensation may return to normal in 18 months.
- **Infection**: Increasing tenderness, increased temperature is a risk of infection. Make sure that your physician has given you antibiotics and that you take your medication as prescribed.

CHAPTER 16
Liposuction

Pain scale: 3 out of 10
Length of Procedure: Variable from 30-180 minutes
Return to Work Time: 3 days

L iposuction is not a weight reduction plan; it is a body sculpting procedure. The ideal candidate is someone at a stable weight, but has specific areas of the body with excess fatty tissue. Many have tried to lose weight to address these problem areas, but have not been successful. A more focused approach of body sculpting is an excellent choice for these patients. For men, these problem areas tend to be the flank (spare tire), chest, or under the chin. For women, the problem areas are lateral thighs (saddle bags), inner thighs, abdomen, back, and upper and lower arm area.

Liposuction is gaining increasing popularity; however, proper patient selection is a key to success. It is one of the most commonly requested procedures and is sometimes used in conjunction with other surgeries. For example, on many Face lifts, there may be liposuction performed around the jaw and chin area. On many tummy tucks, liposuction is performed on the side to shape out the contour. Certain body areas are more amenable to liposuction. Skin tone, elasticity, and the amount of fat to be removed are all key variables for a successful outcome. Your physician will examine your skin and the areas of concern and will be able to predict the outcome of the procedure fairly well.

Defined areas should be selected rather than attempting to reduce fat in the entire body. Liposuction should not be used as a weight loss plan but rather a liposculpting for particular areas. The risk of death from this procedure is 1 in 10,000.

The Procedure

There are several techniques which can be used. The guiding principles are that saline solution mixed with local anesthetic and epinephrine is mixed and injected into the fatty areas to be sculpted. This solution numbs the area, helps to liquefy the fat, and most importantly, constricts the blood vessels to reduce bleeding.

Tumescent technique is where a large volume of fluid is injected into the affected area. Through a small incision, a thin hollow tube (cannula) is inserted into the fatty area, and, like a vacuum, suction is applied, and the fat is sucked out.

A newer technology (power liposuction) combines the tumescent technique with a motorized, vibrating cannula. This combination of techniques can be useful in tougher areas such backs or men's' chests, which require significant fat removal.

Ultrasound liposuction is when a larger cannula is inserted into a bigger incision. The tip of the cannula produces ultrasound waves, which break up the fat into an emulsion. This allows the fat to be more easily removed. A disadvantage is that the tip gets hot, so it has an added risk of burning the skin. The incision in this procedure is also larger than the others to accommodate the ultrasound device. These scars will be slightly larger.

You should discuss with your surgeon which technique he will use to get the best result. There is no right and wrong procedure; this is to provide you with some insight into the different techniques so that you can have a discussion with your surgeon.

On the day of surgery, your surgeon will mark your body in the standing position. Concentric circles will be drawn to indicate where the fat should be removed, and feathered at the edges to create a smooth look. Unlike other procedures where antibiotics may not be necessary, in this case, antibiotics are given intravenously during the surgery to prevent infection.

Recovery Period

That evening at home, you will notice fluid dripping out from the incisions where the cannulae were inserted. Do not be alarmed at the sight of these fluids. Especially with the tumescent technique, it is expected that fluids will seep out for the next 24 hours. This fluid is mixed with blood, but this is normal. It is recommended that you wear old pajamas or cover your bed with old towels to absorb this fluid.

There will be increased swelling for two to three days. On the fourth day, you should be fit into a snug garment, which applies compression to the area that has been liposuctioned. This garment needs to be worn for a six week period. Wearing this garment can be very warm and uncomfortable in the summer; therefore, you should consider having this procedure in the cooler seasons.

Remember that it takes nine months to a year for full healing to occur. Many patients are disappointed in the first few weeks after surgery and ask when the swelling will go down. It takes months for all of the swelling and smoothness to occur; this needs to be explained pre-operatively to avoid disappointment. Even when patients are told not to expect immediate results, they often find it hard to wait. As nine months approaches, patients are happy with their decision to have liposuction.

Myths and Rumors

There are many myths and misconceptions surrounding this procedure. Some people believe that fat will never appear again in the liposculpted area. Others think that fat will accumulate somewhere else in the body. The fact is if you keep at the same weight, the new shape will remain for a long time. If, however, you gain weight, you will gain weight in the sculpted area. Your body fat distribution is predetermined and will go back to the original shape if significant weight is added.

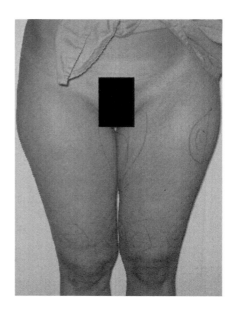

Liposuction Pre-op

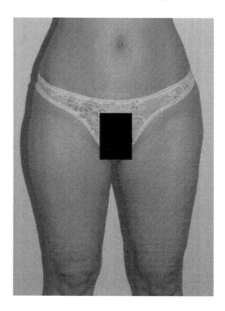

Liposuction Post-Op

Do's and Don'ts

- Do expect some blood tinged fluid to ooze out of the incision site for 1 day.
- Do wear your garment as instructed by your physician. Do be patient and allow it to heal for a year.
- Do have towels and old sheets on your bed to absorb any fluid.
- Do expect numbness over the skin for a few months.
- Do massage the area with moisturizer three times per day.
- Do take showers daily; do not wash by going into a tub.

Complications

Listed below are some possible complications that may occur with this procedure. Your surgeon will review the possible complications with you when you are asked to consent for surgery

- **Infection** may occur even after antibiotics are administered intravenously on the day of surgery. When you get home you should have a prescription for antibiotics. Make sure that you complete the entire bottle.
- **Fat emboli and shock** are the most serious complications typically associated with larger volumes of liposuction. These life threatening complications are rare and usually associated with larger procedures.
- **Irregular scarring or dimpling of the skin:** Some of the skin may appear dimpled or puckered. Much of the irregularities and firmness and numbness will improve over the course of several months up to a year. Some of the dimpling may be permanent and require further liposuction or even fat injection to even out the skin texture.

CHAPTER 17
The Truth About Scars

This chapter applies to any of the chapters you have already read because all procedures involve scarring. Many people think that with today's technology and advances in surgery think that scars are invisible. Plastic surgeons spend a career trying to minimize the scars and have developed experience and techniques to hide the scars but keep in mind that wherever there is a cut, there is a scar. This may sound scary but it s the truth. Several factors can contribute to scarring. Some are controllable by your physician and some are not.

- **Incision placement**: Your surgeon may make the incision in a hidden area. Meticulous placements in hidden places, or areas where there are natural color changes occur are the best locations for an incision. In endoscopic brow lift, for example, the scars are placed in the hairline in between follicles. Face lift incisions are placed inside the ear, behind the ear, or in the scalp, which make them invisible. Incisions for upper lid blepharoplasties are placed at the crease line and are almost undetectable progress in concealing the scars.

- **Technique:** Surgical technique is an important skill that is critical in preventing scar formation. Plastic surgeons are trained in these techniques to minimize scar formation. This is the reason why patients often request a plastic surgeon to repair lacerations, old scars, or wound closures when they are concerned about visible scarring. Plastic surgery technique involves several unique skills, which are part of the training of a plastic surgeon.

- **Skin type:** It is a well known fact that the darker the skin, the more likely the chances of hypertrophic scarring or keloid scarring. Some dark-skinned individuals will know if they are prone to keloid formation. The most important component of scar formation is your genetic make up and your body's ability to heal from an incision. Your history of healing should be discussed with your surgeon as this is one of the best predictors of how your scar will look.

Your surgeon has spent years training for this moment. Often, plastic surgery residents wonder why they are spending years dealing with microvascular surgery connecting blood vessels and nerves if they are planning to perform cosmetic surgeries. This is a requirement for a plastic surgeon, since it is the same high skill level that is required to reconnect a very fine nerve or to make your scar as small as possible. This skill involves a delicate touch to minimize tissue injury while perfectly approximating the deeper layers of the skin. Herein lies one of the plastic surgeons best secrets. By the time the plastic surgeon is closing the outer skin, which is the part you see, it already is held tightly together by deeper layer suturing. In the end, this makes all the difference. The final scar is much finer if there is less tension on the skin. This requires using very fine sutures which are specially designed to minimize scar formation. Even the dressing is important in minimizing scarring. There is a difference in how the body heals in different locations. Areas on the face tend to heal much better than incisions on the back or arms. Incisions in the eyelids or face tend to heal better. Your surgeon can, to a certain degree predict the healing. Incisions behind the ear in the scalp heal with a thick scar. Incisions on the chest or back heal poorly, even with the best surgical technique. The combination of all these components is important to optimize your body's formation of the best scar. It is important to have a discussion with your surgeon regarding what can be done to minimize your scarring.

What you can do to improve the outcome:

- Follow all post operative directions
- On your first post-operative day, your surgeon will remove the sutures. You may be asked to replace steri-strips for several weeks to keep tension off the wound. This will help the scar be finer in the end.
- Depending on how your scar is healing, your surgeon may elect to do one of several things. If it is healing nicely, your surgeon

will advise to follow a routine protocol, such as avoidance of one sun exposure for one full year.

- After applying the steri-strips for six weeks, you can then apply topical Vitamin E to be massaged on the wound three times a day. Scientifically, some people prefer cocoa butter, some Vitamin E. It is not as much the choice of the topical but more the massaging that helps promote better healing and less scar formation.

- If the scar is not healing well, your surgeon may elect to apply a steroid impregnated tape, silicone gel sheets or even inject the scar with a steroid. Remember, it take a full year or healing to really see what the scar will look like. You need to be patient. Think back when you were a child. You may have had a bad scar and now you cannot find it. Statistically, in my practice, many patients are concerned about their scarring for the first few months after surgery. More than 90% of patients find that when they wait a year, they are satisfied with the appearance of their scar and require no further treatment.

- Scar revision: Typically, the preference is to wait nine months to a year to see that the final scar will look like. It is key is to remember that patience is a key factor. The longer you wait, the better the scar will get. Even if the surgeon needs to re-operate, the longer the surgeon waits the better the final result will be.

If the scar is not acceptable after a year what can be done?

There are several choices depending on what caused the scar, how it was closed the first time, and what the scar looks like after a year. Sometimes, a scar caused by blunt trauma can be revised surgically using plastic surgery technique and look fine. Sometimes, incisions are closed in an emergency setting and no attention was paid to detail. Although this was the correct choice at the time, your plastic surgeon may be able to repair the scar later.

Often touch-ups are performed after cosmetic surgery to make the scars look better after a year. These touch-ups are not uncommon in certain procedures, such as tummy tucks. Some scars can be lasered or dermabraded after a year to polish the skin smoother. Another technique is to change the direction of the scar. These procedures are called Z-plasties or flap rotations, the direction of the scar can be changed, which will enable the scar to heal better. Most troubling is what to do with keloid or hypertrophic scarring. There is no right or wrong answer to this problem. Scar revision can be entertained in these patients but one of the risks is that they can scar even worse. For these patients, a conversation is necessary with your surgeon.

CHAPTER 18
Lips and Peri-Oral Procedures

It is not uncommon that after other cosmetic procedures, or as a primary procedure women may want to fill in their smile lines, enhance their lips, or fill in the lines above their lips. As women mature, their lips thin, the fine lines of the upper lip get deeper, and the folds around their mouths deepen as the fat dissipates from these areas. Lip enhancement is gaining popularity even with younger women and those with thin lips.

Lip Augmentation:
Pain scale: 8 out of 10
Procedure length: 30-60 minutes
Return to work: Depends on the procedure

There are different ways to perform lip augmentation each with its pluses and minuses. The quickest in-office procedure is an injection of a filler material such as Collagen, hyaluronic acid (also known as Restylane or hylaform), or autogenous fat. Another product that has been used, but I do not recommend, is hydroxyapetite, also known as radiance. Hydroxyapetite while longer lasting (months or years) can leave visible lumps in the lips. Collagen can be injected right into the lips to give an immediate response. Collagen usually lasts about three months. Restylane is another good product for in-office procedures and can last up to six months.

Procedure
The lips have the greatest number of nerve endings and blocking these nerves can sometimes be painful. Local anesthetic is injected to the nerve of the lips, and a needle is used to inject the filler evenly and slowly. This is a meticulous process with a high degree of patient satisfaction.

Recovery

Immediately after the procedure, your lips will be swollen and your surgeon will give you ice to apply. Continue to place these cold ice compresses on your lips for the first 24 hours. Your lips will continue to swell for two or three days. Don't be alarmed at this swelling. The swelling will come down to its resting place in a two week time period. For the next few months, you will be happy with your lips and you may wish that your surgeon made them fuller. Unlike other body parts, fillers in the lips tend to be resorbed the quickest. This tends to be because of the muscle action of the lips. At this point, patients who like the fuller lips tend to desire a longer lasting procedure. There are several other possible options for lip augmentation: autologous fat injections and permanent lip implants.

Autologous Fat Injection: Fat is harvested from anywhere in the body, processed, then used as filler and injected into lips. Harvesting fat involves selection of a body site such as abdomen or buttocks, administering local anesthetic, and suctioning the fat out in a similar fashion to liposuction, but in smaller volume and more delicately done. Special cannulae and suction devices are used to preserve the viability of the fat. The fat is then re-injected with special cannualae and this fat is used to plump up the lips. A good volume of fat is used to plump up the lips because some of the fat and liquid is resorbed over the next few weeks. Your lips will be more swollen than if you have used Collagen or Restylane® in the past due to this overcompensation. The advantage of the procedure is that it is your own body's material that makes it more natural. The disadvantage is that harvesting the fat is more involved that simply taking filler off the shelf. This process is ideal if you are having liposuction or some other procedure and can combine it with the fat transfer.

Alloderm implants: Alloderm is a product produced by Lifecell, which is processed human skin from cadavers. This processing will allow the skin to be better accepted by your body and remove all cellular components which can cause rejection. Originally, it was hoped that this would yield a long lasting change but over time, this has not been proven. Like most fillers used in the lip, the Alloderm has a variable rate of resorption and may last only several months. The Alloderm comes in freeze-dried packets, which are reconstituted to form sheets, which can then be rolled into different shapes. An incision is made at the ends of the lips and an instrument is used to insert the Alloderm into the patient's lips. The advantage of Alloderm is that it requires only two small, readily available, comes in different sizes and shapes, feels natural , well received by the body, contours very nicely to the body and does not require the surgeon to remove it from the patient's own body. It has not been linked to any transmission of AIDS or Hepatitis. The disadvantage is that it is expensive and patients are sometimes not comfortable with the concept of using cadaver dermis.

Temporalis Fascia: An alternative to Alloderm is to use your own fascia (layer of tough fibrous tissue which surrounds muscles). It can easily be harvested from a well hidden area in your scalp. The incision is well hidden by your hair. The insertion procedure is the same as with Alloderm. The advantage is that this is your own tissue and it feels natural. The disadvantage is that the procedure is more complicated and entails more risk than the Alloderm procedure.

Permanent implants: This requires surgery where an implant is inserted into the lip to increase their size. Gortex is a permanent material that is implanted into the lips. This material can be applied surgically to the upper lip and feels firmer than the natural lip, but will not dissolve over time. The disadvantage is that it will not feel natural, become infected, or protrude out of the lip sometimes requiring surgical removal. Only patients who have not been satisfied with injectables or fat transfers and understand the risks of an implant should consider an implant.

Do's and Don'ts
- Do start with temporary filler to see how you like it before attempting a permanent implant
- Do realize that you will look like a caricature for three days to two weeks
- Don't use silicone in your lips; it can look unnatural and migrate through your body
- Don't do lip augmentation when you have social plans immediately thereafter

Complications

Listed below are some possible complications that may occur with this procedure. Your surgeon will review the possible complications with you when you are asked to consent for surgery

- **Asymmetry:** You may have more swelling on one side of the lip, or have more material deposited in one area which may cause an asymmetric appearance.
- **Resorption:** Unlike anywhere else in the body, the lips tend to resorb filling material faster than anywhere else. One theory is that the material is resorbed in the lips at a faster rate because of the movement of the lip muscles. Patients will need to repeat the procedure to sustain their desired effect when temporary fillers are used.

CHAPTER 19
Facial Contouring: Cheek and Chin Implants

Cheek Implants
Pain Scale: 6 out of 10
Length of time: 60-90 minutes each procedure
Return to Work Time: 1 week

Cheek augmentation is a commonly requested procedure. People who seek this procedure typically feel that their cheeks or face have drooped through the years and lost their youthful appearance. Others who are younger, but who have long-shaped faces, may want to add more prominent looking cheeks. New cheeks here will change the appearance rather than being used to recapture youth.

The Procedure
There are two main ways in which to plump up the cheek area. One way is to insert an implant; the other way is to inject fat into the area. Implants are typically made of a solid silicone material (slapstick) or some other bio-compatible material. An incision is placed inside the mouth underneath the lip. Through this incision, the skin and muscle of the face are peeled off the bone using a special instrument. The opening is enlarged to accommodate the implant which will be placed on top of the cheekbone and secured. There are several methods in which to secure the implant and your surgeon will have his/her preference. The main object is to try and prevent any movement inside the cheek. Depending on the size of the implant, your surgeon can determine the amount of augmentation and prominence. The incision is closed inside the mouth with an absorbable suture. There are no external incisions or visible scars with this procedure. Cheek implants are performed under general anesthesia and require no overnight stay.

There are several complications associated with cheek implants. Any time you insert a foreign object inside the body, you need to worry about infection, extrusion (body pushing the object out), or movement of the implant. These complications, while infrequent, do occur and should be discussed with your surgeon. If you are made aware of possible complications, you will know what symptoms are signs of trouble and you can contact your surgeon.

Recovery Period

When you wake up, your cheeks will be very large and very numb. The reason for this is because local anesthetic has been injected into the surgical site. One of the main nerves (infra-orbital nerve) in your face is now temporarily numb. The sensation will be strange and may somewhat surprising to you. This nerve numbness is akin to a circuit breaker in your home being temporarily shut off. The sensation will return beginning after five hours. Full sensation will not occur for several weeks; it is important that you are aware of the time period so that you are not overly concerned. The next thought you will have is that too large an implant has been placed. There will be swelling over the implant from the surgery which will make it appear more pronounced. You will also notice a small amount of bruising around the cheek area. This swelling and bruising will continue to increase over the next three days but by the fourth day it starts to subside. As the swelling subsides over the next several weeks, the new contour and shape will be more visible.

Sutures have been placed inside your mouth and may feel like dental floss in the pouch between your gums and cheeks. Gargling warm salt water will help the area and reduce the swelling. The sutures will dissolve over the next two weeks, but may be removed by your surgeon earlier if you find them irritating. You will take pain medication for three days as you may experience some discomfort in the cheek area. By day five, you will probably be able to stop using the narcotics and can switch to extra strength Tylenol.

Over the next two-six weeks, the swelling will continue to subside and the discoloration will go away. At six weeks, it will look markedly improved as most of the bruising and swelling has disappeared. The numb sensation should be greatly improved by now. In some people, however, it may take several months to feel normal sensation in the cheeks.

Patients are usually checked by the surgeon during the first two weeks and again after several months to see the final results.

Complications

Listed below are some possible complications that may occur with this procedure. Your surgeon will review the possible complications with you when you are asked to consent for surgery

- **Infection**: Make sure that you take your antibiotic to minimize the possibility of infection.
- **Loss of sensation**: The infraorbital nerve can be stretched or injured during this procedure. This is usually numb for the first few weeks and then sensation returns.
- **Extrusion or displacement**: The implant may move or change positions, or can be extruded into the oral cavity.

Chin Augmentation

Pain Scale: 8 out of 10
Length of Procedure: Less than one hour
Return To Work Time: One week

This procedure augments or increases a weak or small chin. Often, this procedure is done in patients who are dissatisfied with the balance of their lower face. It is often performed in concert with a rhinoplasty or liposuction of the neck or jaw area. A simple way to determine whether you are a good candidate is to take a photo of your side profile. Draw a vertical line from your upper lip perpendicularly straight down toward your chin. If your face is in balance, the chin will come close to touching this vertical line. In women, the chin may be slightly behind this line and be appropriate. In men, where a more prominent is considered handsome, the chin should come close to or touch the vertical line. If there is space between the chin and this line, one could consider a chin implant.

Chin implants are typically made out of a solid silicone although they come in a variety of materials. This surgery is done under light sedation with local anesthetic placed where the implant will be positioned. The incision can be placed either inside the mouth or underneath the chin. If the incision is made inside the lip, a small pocket is made over the chin bone and the implant is placed meticulously into this pocket. The main advantage of the technique is that there are no visible scars. The disadvantage is that there is a higher rate of implant infection since it must go through the oral cavity. Alternatively, an external incision allows the implant to be placed through the skin rather than the oral cavity. Introduction through the skin has less risk of infection as compared to your mouth. This procedure, however, leaves a small scar under the chin which will usually heal inconspicuously. You and your surgeon will discuss the options and decide which procedure is right for you.

Some patients ask why they have not heard any controversy about using silicone in chin implants. Breast implants are basically balloons filled with liquid silicone. The concern for breast implants is that if the implant ruptures, the liquid silicone is released into the body. The controversial issue is whether or not this released silicone can cause immune problems. The silicone used for chin implants is a solid and does not the same concern as the liquid breast implants. Therefore, there has been no controversy about using silicone chin implants.

Post-Operative Recovery

After surgery, the lower lip will be numb for several hours due to the local anesthetic. This will feel similar to what you would feel after a dental anesthetic is applied. As the anesthesia wears off, you will experience some discomfort at the surgical site. When you get home, you should have the pain medication ready and take it before the numbing wears off from the local anesthetic. Follow the instructions you have been provided. Also, take the antibiotic that was prescribed to reduce the risk of infection. Take the antibiotics on the same day you arrive home and make sure that you finish the course.

The complications for the chin implant procedure are the same as the cheek with the addition of possible numbness in the mental nerves under the chin. This loss of sensation is temporary and should return in a few weeks.

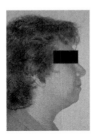   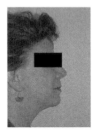

Chin Augmentation Pre-op   Chin Augmentaton Post-op

PART III
Non-Surgical Procedures

There are many other options other than surgery to make your appearance more youthful. In recent years, there has been technology such as lasers, which have advanced, and fillers, such as Collagen, Botox®, Juvederm ® and Restylane®. We will be discussing these office-based procedures that are inexpensive relaitve to surgery, but not as long lasting. People who are not yet ready for surgery, or seek refinement after surgery are usually very satisfied with these procedures. These are more maintenance procedures that can keep people looking youthful, healthy, and not overdone. We will review with you the most common non-surgical procedures. There are an ever increasing number of these procedures and they are gaining popularity. You will likely have read about many of these options in magazines or have seen them on talk shows

CHAPTER 20
Lasers

Laser technology is based on a theory developed by Einstein. The word laser is an acronym for LIGHT AMPLIFICATION BY STIMLULATED EMISSION OF RADIATION. All lasers are built with three basic elements: reflective mirrors, an energy source, and some laser medium. This medium is typically made of a gas, which, when stimulated with electricity, emits photons of one wavelength in a powerful beam. By manipulating the wavelength the laser creates, only certain elements in the skin are treated. Several unique properties of the laser such as its intensity and wavelength allow it to be a unique tool in creating cosmetic improvements. Some lasers can selectively destroy unwanted pigments, hairs, or veins without injuring surrounding structures. Through technology changes and advancements, lasers have improved over the years. Similar to breakthroughs in other technologies, lasers have become smaller, easier to use, more effective and less expensive. They have become a popular option for those patients who desire minor improvements or are not yet ready for surgery.

Lasers are an excellent treatment option for the following skin conditions:
- Skin rejuvenation
- Red spots and broken capillaries (red lines on the face)
- Hair removal
- Tattoo removal
- Vein removal
- Aging and brown spot removal
- Acne scar revision
- Rosacea
- Birthmarks

There are two major classes of lasers ablative and non ablative.

Ablative lasers

Ablative lasers heat up the water in the skin which causes a burn. The skin becomes reddened, weepy, scabby, and swollen for approximately two weeks. Redness may persist for months, which is the major downside of this type of procedure. The advantage of these lasers is since they obliterate the surface of the skin, it can create a dramatic change. The disadvantage of using this laser is that it is painful, has a longer recovery time, requires anesthesia or sedation, and is more invasive than other types of lasering. Ablative lasers are used for removal of fine lines, often in conjunction with a Face lift. There are two types of ablative lasers: Carbon Dioxide and Erbium lasers. People thought that the Carbon Dioxide laser would be a panacea, but patients realized that their skin remained red for many months. To resume their normal activity, they were required to wear concealing make up. A newer technology was the Erbium laser. This is also ablative, but less destructive and doesn't go as deep as the Carbon Dioxide laser. As one would expect, however, there is slightly less improvement with this laser. Some physicians will use a combination of each laser to get the best result with the least downtime.

Non-Ablative Lasers

The light shines through the outer layer of skin and targets structures such as the unwanted hairs, brown spots, or red spots without leaving visible marks and blistering on the outer skin. There are many different lasers that are used for specific indications. A KTP laser is used for redness of the skin (telangectacia) and Yag laser is used to target dark hair follicles for hair removal. Other lasers are used for increasing Collagen for fine line improvement. These lasers tend to be much less painful than the ablative lasers. Patients have said that these lasers feel similar to a rubber band snapping you. To avoid damage to the eyes, you will be asked to wear protective eyewear during your laser procedure. These glasses are a necessary precaution for all laser procedures, even if the treatment is not near the face or eyes.

While lasers have made tremendous progress, many patients have come to think of them as panaceas and replacements for plastic surgery.

For many procedures, lasering may be a viable option but it does not replace the need for surgery in many cases. It cannot get rid of thick scars, deep wrinkles, or droopy skin.

The Ablative Procedures

Pre-operatively, if you are having work performed in the peri-oral area (around the mouth), you may be given an anti viral medication such as Valtrex or Zovirax to prevent cold sores. 80% of the population has had an outbreak of a cold sore (herpes) at one time in their life. A herpetic outbreak may occur after a laser treatment, which is why the anti-viral agent is prescribed.

Ablative lasering is performed under sedation on an outpatient basis. In addition to the sedation, a local anesthetic is applied to numb the skin. When you wake up from the procedure, you will see redness in the skin. As the local anesthetic wears off, you will experience stinging in the area. You will need to take the antibiotics and pain medications as prescribed.

Day One

You should shower with cool water to gently rinse the skin. Dry with a soft, clean, white towel and apply the any topical ointments that your physician has prescribed. Some will prescribe an antibiotic, some use anti-inflammatory cream and some use a moisturizer such as Aquaphor. There is no one-favored method; your physician may try several ways to make you feel comfortable.

Weeks Two and Three

Your face will become crusted and begin to ooze. These are normal effects of this procedure. Continue with the daily showering and application of creams. After seven to ten days, the crusting will fall off and skin will be red underneath. The new skin will be smooth and red, but over weeks and months to come, the redness will fade. After about 12-14 days, depending on healing, you can use cover up make up and resume normal activities,

Non-Ablative Lasering

This procedure is much less painful—usually a topical cream is applied about thirty minutes prior to the procedure. Some procedures do not require any anesthesia and the patient can go through the procedure without major discomfort. At the time of the procedure, the cream is removed and the skin feels numb. There are several techniques to cool the skin to reduce pain, redness, and blistering. Some lasers use a cool cryogen spray and others use cool tip with cooling gel. There are several lasers on the market which feel different to patients. In general, the skin is cooled and the laser beam goes through the outer layer of skin to the layer underneath to correct the area of concern. Of all the procedures, the hair removal and vein removal are the most uncomfortable. The removal of light brown spots is fairly painless. Some patients have reported that certain laser procedures, such as skin rejuvenation, feels like a rubber band snapping on the skin.

After the procedure, a thin later of hydrocortisone cream is applied to help reduce any redness. If the skin is warm, a cold ice pack may be applied. Redness may persist for several hours after the procedure. When the laser treatment is over, there is minimal discomfort. You can resume normal activity immediately. For procedures involving treatment of leg veins, the patient must wear support hose for two or three days to constrict the area. These support hose are not painful, but some patients feel uncomfortable wearing them, especially in the summer months. They will, however, improve the result of the vein removal.

Managing expectations

It is very important that your surgeon manage your expectation. These lasers treatments require several treatments for a successful result. Although there is very little down time, on average, it takes three to five treatments to really see results.

CHAPTER 21
Fillers, Peels, and Botox®

You have probably heard a lot about fillers, but what are they? These materials are injected into the skin to plump up fine lines and reduce their appearance. As we age, a combination of agents such as sun damage, gravity, thinning of the skin, and years of muscle activity will lead to the appearance of fine lines and wrinkles. Common areas for these wrinkles or smile lines are the corners of the eyes, around the lips, on the chin between the eyes and on the forehead. The good news is that there are many new products that are relatively simple procedures which can reduce the appearance of these lines. Most fillers will temporarily fill in these areas so that the lines are not noticeable. The skin appears smoother and the lines are significantly diminished for several months. Pharmaceutical companies are constantly improving the fillers; making them last longer, have less allergic reactions, and look more natural. Your physician may use different filling agents depending on the depth of the wrinkle.

Collagen

Collagen has been used as a filler agent for many years. Originally, it was derived from the dermis of a cow. Five percent of patients used to get allergic reactions to this substance and allergy testing would need to be done prior to treatment. There is a new Collagen (Cosmoplast®), which is derived from a human source. Allergy testing is not required on this substance. This substance is mixed with lidocaine so that when injected, it numbs the skin. This material is excellent for reduction of fine "smile" lines, such as those around the lips and chin. The lines are not deep and can easily be treated by this filler.

The advantage of this material is that is not painful, heals well, is relatively inexpensive, and looks great. Collagen is a very fine substance and is best used for fine superficial lines. The downside is that the result is short term and only lasts three months. After your injection, you will typically feel small lumps and bumps. The reason you have these bumps is because there is swelling around the injection sites. Also, the physician will purposely inject more collagen than is needed for an overcorrection because some of it is absorbed into the skin. If the surgeon over-injects slightly to compensate for this, you will have a more natural, longer lasting effect.

This procedure usually takes fifteen minutes. The area is cleaned and a very fine needle is used to inject the Collagen. There is minimal discomfort similar to a mosquito bite. The small needle in inserted many times into the skin to inject tiny bits of Collagen into the fine lines. You may use a cool ice pack to reduce any bruising and swelling which may occur after the procedure.

Right after the procedure, you will notice lumps and bumps and may be surprised or concerned about the immediate result. Over two or three days, it may swell or bruise even more. You may apply cover up makeup, shower, and resume normal activities. Over the next twelve days, the look will soften and you will be satisfied with the result.

Radiance®

Radiance® is the trade name for a substance called Hydroxyapatite. Hydroxyapatite is a porous, granular material. It is another injectable that has gained popularity in the market within the last few years. It is made of the same material that makes up coral reefs. This substance gained popularity because these Hydroxapatite treatments last for years. The only solution to this was to cut out the pellets. Hydroxyapatite is best used for deep folds around the nose (lasolabial folds). I don't recommend it for small lines around the lips because it has been reported that patients feel small pebble like particles where the substance is injected. You should discuss the pros and cons of this treatment with your physician.

This procedure is performed in an out patient office. You will receive a local anesthetic first. The substance in injected and you will see an immediate response.

Restylane®

Restylane® is a trade name for a product that contains Hyaluronic Acid. This clear odorless soft substance is made from sugars which are naturally occurring in the body. Hyaluronic Acid is found in joints and functions as a cushion and lubricant for tissues in the body. Adding this substance to wrinkles will allow a more youthful and younger appearance. This substance is free of animal proteins, which limits the risk of allergic reaction. No pre testing of this product is necessary. Restylane® is newer to the market, integrates into the tissue naturally, and lasts approximately six months. It also feels soft like the skin and is easy to inject. Patient satisfaction is high with this product. Restylane® is thicker in consistency than Collagen. It is used to provide volume and fullness to moderate wrinkles rather than fine lines. Typically, Restylane® is used for lines in the face. If the patient wants a smoother look or wants a more dramatic change, more Restylane® can be added at any time.

This substance does not come prefabricated with a local anesthetic. You will be given a local anesthetic prior to the Restylane® injection. This will numb the area; a cold ice pack may be applied to prevent swelling and bruising. The area is then injected with a fine bead of material. There may be multiple injections at the site if necessary to fill in the lines. Patient satisfaction with this treatment is very high.

After the procedure, there may be some swelling and bruising and some redness at the injection site. This redness and bruising will resolve in two or three days. Immediately after the procedure, an ice pack may be applied to cool and compress the area. You can resume normal activities immediately after the procedure.

Autogenous Fat Transfer

Autogenous Fat transfer is the removal and processing of fat from one part of your body and reinjection into another. Since this is your own bodies' material, it is safe and poses no risk of allergic reaction. The advantage of this procedure is that it's longer lasting, more natural and has an extremely high patient satisfaction rate. There is also an abundance of fat in the body which is readily available for transfer. The disadvantage is that this takes more time and is more involved than a simple injection of Restylane® or Collagen. In my experience, fat transfer can have long lasting effects. It is possible that some of the fat can remain viable for up to several years. If the fat is removed and processed meticulously, there is an increased survival rate. Fat transfers are most commonly used to fill in deep lines in the nasolabial folds or contour irregularities in the body.

This procedure involves injection of local anesthetic combined with salt water solution into the site from where the fat will be harvested. The solution is left in place for ten minutes to numb the area. A small incision is made in the skin and a cannula or small tube is inserted into the area. Fat and the fluid are aspirated out through the tube and processed. It is then transferred to smaller syringes and injected into the wrinkles and folds. After this procedure, there will be marked swelling in the area where the fat was injected. Fat is typically removed from your buttocks, thighs, or abdomen. This area will have a small suture in it where the cannula was inserted. It will also be bruised and swollen after the procedure. Over two or three days, the area where the fat was injected will feel swollen and you may be worried that too much fat was injected. You must remember that much of this is swelling is fluid and edema from the surgery. Over a two week period, the swelling will subside and the bruising will fade. In six weeks, it will feel like your natural skin and face but without the deep lines or wrinkles.

Juvederm®

Juvederm® is a newer product which is an injectable form of hyaluronic acid. Similar to Restylane®, Juvederm® is a clear, colorless substance which is injected into the skin to reduce the appearance of wrinkles and folds. You will be given a local anesthetic prior to the injection to numb the area. A cold ice pack may be applied to prevent swelling and bruising. The area is injected with a fine thread of Juvederm®. Depending on the depth of the wrinkle or fold, it may be necessary to administer multiple injections at the site to fill in the lines. Patient satisfaction with this treatment is very high.

After the procedure, there may be some swelling and bruising and some redness at the injection site. This redness and bruising will resolve in two or three days. Immediately after the procedure, an ice pack may be applied to cool and compress the area. Any bruising will subside in a few days.

After the procedure, you should avoid strenuous exercise, extensive sun or heat exposure and alcoholic beverages. Otherwise, all normal activities may be resumed immediately after the treatment.

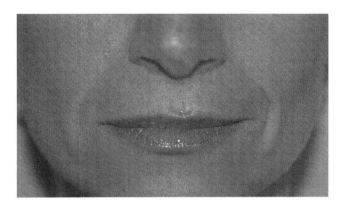

Pre-injection

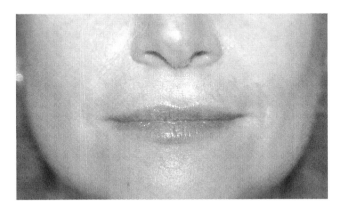

Post—injection

Botox®

Botox ® is one of the most common procedures for eliminating lines in the forehead, crow's feet, or lines between the eyes. It can also be used in other areas of the face such as banding in the neck. Cosmetic surgeons use it for facial lines and spasms of the facial muscles, and excessive sweating in the armpit or palm.

What is Botox®? It is a substance derived from the toxin expressed from the bacteria that causes botulism poisoning. It works by paralyzing muscles and has been used in medicine for decades. It was used to treat muscular spasms for a variety of diseases. As muscles are paralyzed and weakened, the wrinkles in the skin fade if they were not too deep. Many patients are amazed at this process. If the wrinkles are deep and have been present for many years, you may need a filler to eliminate the wrinkles. But, for most fine wrinkles, the Botox® is sufficient. Botox®, if administered correctly by a qualified physician, is considered extremely safe. Keep in mind that there are no shortcuts or discounts with Botox®. The drug must be purchased by a high grade pharmacy. One vial containing 100 units of Botox® costs almost five hundred dollars. If you see Botox® advertised for discounted rates, this is some cause of concern. Either the Botox® may be over diluted, stored for an extended period, or purchased from a questionable source. Any of these three options will lead to a discounted price, but one should questions the results and safety. Botox® purchased from a non-reliable source could be lethal.

Botox® treatment is temporary, lasting approximately three months. Patient satisfaction with Botox® is extremely high and the vast majority of patients seek this procedure again. It is not critical for patients to come like clockwork every three months. Some patients see their lines and wrinkles eventually return and will then seek another Botox® treatment.

The Procedure
This procedure takes fifteen minutes. The skin is cleaned with alcohol, a cool compress may be applied to decrease the pinch of the needles as well as decrease bruising. The Botox® is injected with a tiny needle in the area that you seek to improve. After the injection, a cool compress is applied to reduce any bruising. Similar to tiny mosquito bites, you may see fine drops of blood or swelling. By the time you get home, it is likely to be unnoticeable. Rarely, someone will get bruising, which will subside over the course of several days.

The optimal use of Botox® is enough to eliminate the lines but not so much that there is a loss of facial expression. We have all seen patients who have had too much Botox® injected and their face looks frozen. There is a careful balance creating the cosmetic improvement while avoiding an unnatural look. Often, patients will point to a line right at their brow and want those removed; most times, you are best to leave those alone. Botox® injected too close to the eyebrow can create a droopy look; this is counterproductive to what you are trying to achieve. Botox® can be injected on the side of the eyes near the crow's feet to create an elevated brow look and soften the lines. Botox® can be adjusted over time to get the optimal results. This depends on a combination of the dosing and the result.

How long does it take for the results to take effect? Over the first three days, you will start to notice lessening of the lines. It evens out over the next several days. Many patients think that it did not work over the first few days. Optimal benefit is noticed at two weeks after the treatment. It is not uncommon for patients to want more Botox® in the first week after treatment. They feel that it is not working well or not all of their wrinkles are eliminated. It is important to note that the full effect will not be noticeable for two weeks. In the initial Botox® treatment, it is better for your physician to be conservative. He will record the actual doses used, take note your results, and adjust future doses accordingly. After two weeks, it may be necessary for a touch up by adding a bit more Botox® to get the optimal effect. It is better to use less Botox® and add more if necessary that to use too much and create a droopy look.

What happens if your eyebrow does get droopy? Do not panic; this effect will wear off over the next few weeks. You must notify your physician so that he/she will administer fewer units of Botox® on your next treatment.

CHAPTER 22
Chemical Peels, Dermabrasion, And Microdermabrasion

Peels, Dermabrasion, and Microdermabrasion are procedures that are based on a common principle. All three procedures use different techniques to remove the outer layer of skin, allowing new skin to grow and replace it. The new skin is smoother and more youthful than the old skin that was shed. Each procedure uses a different technique which will be described below.

If a patient has taken the drug Accutane within the past year, they are not a candidate for skin resurfacing because of the increased risk of scarring.

Peels
Chemical peels cause a predictable injury to the superficial layer of the skin, causing it to shed. New, healthy skin will grow in its place, which results in improved tone and texture. Peels are solutions that gently burn the outer layer of skin. It may flake off and newer healthier skin grows in its place to create a smoother surface. Chemical peels come in a variety of different chemicals and concentrations. Different combinations of time and concentration will determine the outcome. Some chemicals used as peeling compounds include: Glycolic acid, Trichloroacetic acid (TCA), and Salicylic acid. These chemicals are used in different concentrations depending on the physician and the desired effect.

Peels do not tighten or lift skin, but may improve the quality of the skin. Lighter peels can be used for some improvement in patients who do not want lasering or surgery. It is used for very fine lines and may improve the texture of the skin. The peeled skin grows back over the course of two weeks and creates a smoother, fresher look. Unfortunately, the new look is not permanent and will only last three or four months.

Although peels do not create a dramatic change, they are still chemicals and needed to be handled appropriately. It is important to be treated under a physician's supervision to prevent complications. These chemicals may burn the skin too much if used improperly. Excessive burning will result in scarring rather than the desired look of new, smooth skin. To prevent complications, make sure that you are treated by an experienced professional working under the direction of a physician.

Dermabrasion

This is another technique used to rejuvenate skin. A mechanical wheel is used to grind down the outer layer of skin. This allows the new cells underneath to be stimulated to grow a new outer layer of skin. This new layer is finer and smoother than the old skin. This is used for fine to medium lines as well as acne scarring. This process is similar to the skin rejuvenation which occurs after carbon dioxide lasering.

Advantages of Dermabrasion vs. Carbon Dioxide Lasering: The redness caused by lasering may last many months. In dermabrasion, the redness subsides quicker, in approximately two months. Cover-up make-up may be used in both of these procedures but the recovery time is quicker with Dermabrasion. Dermabrasion will make a marked improvement after one treatment, but several treatments may be required for the desired effect.

Disadvantage: This procedure requires a high degree of skill by the surgeon and experience in using this equipment. If it is done too superficially, there is not enough significant change. If it is done too deeply, scarring may result. If done correctly, patients are usually very satisfied with their result.

Procedure

This procedure is performed in an outpatient setting or physician's office. You will receive sedation and a local anesthetic. The skin is cleaned with antiseptic solution and the dermabrader is applied to the outer layers of skin. A dermabrader has a grinding bit made of micro wire brushes or polishing stone. The skin is held taut and the outer layer is sanded away. It is performed deeper in areas where the lines or scars are more pronounced and feathered out to blend in with healthier looking skin so there is no obvious demarcation. Depending on the amount of skin that needs to be dermabraded, this procedure may take between thirty minutes and one hour. Upon completion, your surgeon will apply topical ointment such as a moisturizer. The sedation will wear off but you will have little discomfort because the local anesthetic is still in effect. Over the next four to five hours, the local anesthetic will wear off and you will feel burning where the skin was abraded. You will be given pain medication that you should take when you get home even before you experience any discomfort. You should take a prescribed pain medication over the next two to three days to minimize discomfort. After three days, you may take extra strength Tylenol as needed.

If you are being treated in the peri-oral area, prior to your procedure, you will be required to take an anti-viral medication like Zovirax® if you have any history of herpes (cold sores).

Day Two to Four

Over the next few days, the area will become scabby, dripping, and crusty and you will think that something has gone wrong. This is part of the normal healing process and should not be cause for alarm. On day two, you should shower with warm water and a light spray with a gentle shampoo on your hair. Pat dry with a clean towel and apply with the ointment that was prescribed by your physician. Some physicians prescribe a topical antibiotic ointment to decrease infections but 10% of the population has an allergic reaction to the antibiotic. Other physicians prescribe only a moisturizer such as Aquaphor. In any event, it is important to shower once to twice a day. You will also be given an oral antibiotic which you must take for the entire course to minimize skin infection.

The Following Week

On day seven to twelve the scabs will fall off and the skin underneath will be smoother and pinkish. Cover-up make-up may be applied at day twelve. Over the next few weeks, you will see the redness subside and the contour of the skin start to improve.

Retin A®

Retin A® is the shortened name for Retinoic Acid. This has been used effectively applied to the outer layer of skin. It thickens the deeper layers of skin which gives a healthier looking complexion and in some instances will improve the appearance of fine lines around the eyes. Although the results are minimal, they are real improvements for many patients. You have to have realistic expectations if you use Retin A®. Results will not be noticed for at least six weeks. When they are noticed, the results are very subtle. Like in other treatments, it is important to manage a patient's expectations.

Retin A® is fabricated in different strengths by different pharmaceutical companies. Physicians typically start out with a lower concentration. You will be asked to apply a thin layer of it in the evening around the eyes. At first, apply it on Monday, Wednesday, and Friday. If there is no redness or sensitivity, you may then apply it every day. If you have no reaction, your physician will prescribe a higher strength to maximize the effects of the medication. On the morning after applying it, you may use moisturizer. If you go into the sun, you must use sunscreen to avoid burning the area.

Many people spend a lot of money for over the counter cosmetics which include Retin A®. The truth is that the concentration of Retin A® in these products is too low to have any long-term clinical effects. Some of the products may feel nice to the touch, or provide good moisturizing, but will have no impact on fine lines or wrinkles.

Microdermabrasion

Microdermabrasion is a simple procedure which should not be confused with Dermabrasion. Microdermabrasion is a very popular non surgical treatment for skin rejuvenation. It is used to help reduce fine lines and acne scarring by stimulating the production of skin cells and Collagen. Typically, your physician will use a hand piece which sprays out fine crystals onto the skin. The process is similar to sandblasting or polishing. These crystals will gently remove the outer superficial layer of damaged skin. Each procedure requires between thirty minutes to an hour and is typically what is referred to as a "lunchtime procedure."

No anesthesia is required; there is little risk or discomfort, and no real downtime associated with this procedure.

As with any other cosmetic procedures, managing patient expectations is an important consideration. Microdermabrasion is not an aggressive procedure and as such, may produce only minor improvements over many treatments. It does not have the risks of pigment changes or scarring which are possible with Dermabrasion or other more invasive procedures.

CHAPTER 23
What's On The Horizon?

Medicine is a quickly evolving field. There are always new drugs, technology, and procedures being developed and evaluated. Those of you who follow these developments will read about the newest ideas in magazines or see them on television. It is important for you to understand that while the frontiers of plastic surgery are exciting, there is a lot of fine tuning necessary to ensure that a procedure is safe and effective. It is common for patients to want to be first in line to try out a new technology or procedure, once they have heard about it. This may not be the wisest move when it comes to medical treatments. There is a steep learning curve with new equipment and procedures. Although companies spend a fortune on advertising new equipment or instruments, it is important that your physician become experienced in using it before we would recommend getting in line.

Many procedures are in development now and could be the standard of care, while others will not succeed. Some will result in complications which are unexpected but take years to unfold. Take all of these new things with caution and speak to your physician about his experience before trying out a new procedure. You don't always have to be the first person to try these new things. Sometimes, it is better to err on the side of caution and sit on the sidelines for a while.

Listed below are just some of the procedures and technology on the horizon. We do not recommend all of these items—this is just a compilation of some newer developments which you may have heard of recently.

Laser technology
Lasers have advanced at rapid rates. Lasers now come in smaller units which are affordable with increased safety and efficacy. One newer

technique which uses radiofrequency not light to melt fat and change contouring on the face. Radiofrequency use is a relative newcomer to the cosmetic field. While some proponents tout it as a wonderful thing, others have found that it is more painful to the patient. This has required further investigation and refinement before it becomes the gold standard. Others have found it to have unexpected complications. There are other lasers in development.

Threading

Thread is used to pull the skin up and sutured in place. The thread pulls up skin taut and knots are placed in the hairline. This is used recently for facial rejuvenation in patients with minimal skin laxity. The advantage is that it is less invasive, heals quickly, and is hidden. This technique is relatively simple to perform and less expensive. The disadvantage is that it cannot be used for patients with excess skin, and can leave puckering in the skin.

Fat

People have been pulling skin tighter and tighter, then realize that the patient still looks old. Now, autogenous fat transfers are being used instead of a Face lift. These fat injections can fill in wrinkles and creases in areas where the fat has thinned.

Endoscopic surgery

This is being pushed to its limits to get smaller and smaller incisions with less invasion. Instruments are also getting smaller and smaller. The advantage of endoscopic technique is less skin cutting with decreased scarring and numbness. The disadvantage is that the surgeon cannot visualize the area as well, therefore making it more challenging to get perfect results. Also, results may not be as long lasting. This procedure cannot be used in patients who desire a significant change. Endoscopic surgery has grown in popularity in brow lifting, breast implants, and forehead lifting.

Face transplant

This is a procedure using donor body parts such as ears, skin, bone, and muscle, which can be transplanted from one person to another. The ethical and moral issues of this procedure are being debated. This procedure was performed recently on a woman who was the victim of trauma. The success of the procedure will need to be followed over several years to gauge its success.

CHAPTER 24
Wrapping It Up

After reading this guide, you have been exposed to many trade secrets and information that you may not have known before. You should now be able to understand your procedure, ask educated questions in your consultation, and be less intimidated with the entire process. As was mentioned earlier, this book is not meant to be a quick read. If you proceed with having a procedure, you should refer to it at the different points in the process. Re-read the consultation section right before you go and meet your surgeon. Understand the different options before signing a consent form. Refer often to the recovery process section for your specific procedure; this information may allay your fears when you notice something a few days after the procedure.

We also hope after reading this book, that you understand that cosmetic procedures do have risks. There are very small complications rates associated with every one of the procedures we described. There are many different variables which can lead to a complication or unexpected event. Your role in this process is to control as many variables as you can to reduce that risk and improve your outcome. Also remember that there are no guarantees but with knowledge, you will have more control over your outcome.

Good luck in pursuing a more beautiful you.

GLOSSARY

Abdominoplasty: A surgical procedure done to flatten your abdomen by removing extra fat and skin, and tightening muscles in your abdominal wall. This procedure is commonly referred to as a tummy tuck.

Arnica: A homeopathic medication used in China for centuries. It comes in pill form and topical cream. It is used pre and post operatively to reduce bruising.

Beta-hydroxy acid: An oil-soluble exfoliant derived from fruit and milk sugars that is commonly found in skin-care products. Beta-hydroxy acid is used to treat wrinkles, blackheads, and photoaging. Salicylic acid is an example of a beta-hydroxy acid.

Blepharoplasty: A primarily cosmetic surgical procedure that reduces bagginess from lower eyelids and raises drooping upper eyelids. The procedure involves the removal of excess skin, muscle, and underlying fatty tissue.

Breast augmentation: A surgical procedure done to increase breast size.

Breast reduction: A surgical procedure done to reduce breast size.

Botox®: A substance derived from botulinum toxin that works by preventing nerve impulses from reaching the muscle, causing the muscle to relax.

Bromelain: An active ingredient found in fresh pineapple and has been found to help decrease swelling and bruising. Bromelain in tablet form may be purchased in vitamin or nutrition shops.

Brow lift: A surgical procedure in which the skin of the forehead and eyebrows is tightened to eliminate sagging eyebrows or correct frown lines in the forehead.

Cheek/Chin Augmentation: A surgical procedure in which implants are placed in the cheeks or chin to improve bone structure and support sagging, soft tissues.

Chemical peel: A process in which a chemical solution is applied to the skin to remove dead skin cells and stimulate the production of new layer of regenerated skin. Chemical peel is an effective treatment for wrinkles caused by sun damage, mild scarring, and certain types of acne.

Collagen: The major structural proteins in the skin that give the skin its strength and resilience.

Crow's Feet: The fine lines found around the eyes. They are often caused by sun exposure and aging; however, smoking also contributes to their formation.

Dermabrasion: A facial sanding technique used to treat deep scars and wrinkles, raised scar tissue, and some severe cases of cystic acne. Top layers of skin are "sanded" off with a high-speed rotating brush or a diamond-coated wheel stimulating the production of a new layer of skin.

Dermis: The middle layer of the skin; the dermis is a complex combination of blood vessels, hair follicles, and sebaceous (oil) glands.

Deviated septum: A condition in which the septum (the wall inside the nose that divides it into two sides) is not located in the middle of the nose where it should be. The condition is commonly treatable with surgery.

Epidermis: The outer layer of the skin. The epidermis is also the thinnest layer, responsible for protecting you from the harsh environment. The epidermis is made up of five layers.

Eye lift: See blepharoplasty

Face lift: See rhytidectomy

Facial Reconstruction: Complex surgical procedure to repair or reconstruct facial features in victims of cancer, facial trauma, and birth defects. Reconstruction often involves the skin, muscles, and nerves.

Fascia: A type of strong connective tissue that is found under the skin. Used during Face lift surgery and other procedures for longer lasting effects. This product is made from human donor tissue.

Filler Injections: Commonly referred to as "plumping agents." Most common fillers are Collagen, a gel like substance derived from purified animal tissue, and fat, which is harvested from the patient's thigh or abdomen. These agents are injected under the skin to plump up facial areas or "fill" wrinkled areas (see also Botox®)

Forehead Lift: Surgery to minimize forehead lines and wrinkles, and to elevate brows to reduce lid drooping.

Gynecomastia: Excessive development of the breast tissue in a male.

Hematoma: A collection of blood that may form after a surgical procedure and causes pain and swelling.

Hypertrophic scar: A raised and red scar which does not resolve normally and sometimes requires a corrective procedure.

Keloid scar: A type of scar that continues to grow beyond the site of an injury. This type of scar is caused by too much Collagen forming while the skin is being repaired. The tendency to develop keloid scars is genetic.

Juvederm®: An injectable form of Hyaluronic acid which is injected to fill in lines and wrinkles.

Laser resurfacing: Light beams vaporize top layers of the skin to lessen the appearance of wrinkles, scars, birthmarks, or to generally resurface facial skin.

Lip Augmentation: A procedure done to improve deflated, drooping, or sagging lips, correct their symmetry or to reduce fine lines and wrinkles around them. This is often done through injections or implants.

Lipoplasty: See liposuction.

Liposuction: A cosmetic procedure in which a special instrument called a cannula is used to break up and suck out fat from the body. This procedure is also known as lipoplasty.

Mammoplasty: Any reconstructive or cosmetic surgical procedure that alters the size or shape of the breast.

Mastectomy: The surgical removal of part or the entire breast. This is commonly performed in patients with breast cancer.

Mastopexy: Also called a breast lift, this procedure removes excess skin in order to lift up sagging or drooping breasts.

Mephyton: Also known as Vitamin K, a key component in the blood clotting process.

Microdermabrasion: A mini-peeling procedure with minimal risk of scarring that is done by projecting aluminum micro-crystals onto the skin to simulate growth of new skin.

Otoplasty: A surgical procedure of the ear where protruding or deformed ears can be "pinned back" by reshaping the cartilage.

Platysma: The second supportive layer of muscle.

Ptosis: The drooping of a body part, especially the eyelids or the breasts.

Restylane®: A filling agent used to improve fine lines and wrinkles

Retinol: A derivative of Vitamin A commonly found in many skin care creams.

Rhinoplasty: Commonly referred to as a nose job, this procedure enhances or changes the appearance of the nose. Cartilage and bone are reshaped and reconstructed and excess bone or cartilage may be removed.

Rhytidectomy: Commonly called a Face lift, this surgical procedure is done to eliminate the sagging, drooping, and wrinkled skin of the face and neck.

Salicylic acid: See beta-hydroxy acid

Scar revision: Procedures to help minimize visible facial scars

Sedation: Medically induced process which causes patients to become drowsy and unaware. Depending on the level and type of anesthesia, patients may be "lightly sedated" or "heavily sedated".

Skin resurfacing: Removal of the outer layer of the skin using abrasion, chemicals, or a laser, resulting in smoother and less wrinkled skin

Suture: The stitches used to hold tissue together or to close a wound.

ABOUT THE AUTHORS
Anthony N. LaBruna, M.D., F.A.C.S.

D r. LaBruna received his Medical Degree from Weill Cornell Medical College with honors in Research. He is also a member of the Alpha Omega Alpha Honor Society. He completed a residency in Plastics and Reconstructive Surgery at The Mount Sinai Medical Center where he served as Chief Resident. He also completed a residency in Otolaryngology—Head and Neck Surgery at Manhattan Eye, Ear and Throat Hospital where he served as Chief Surgical Resident. He is dually board certified in Plastic and Reconstructive Surgery and Otolaryngology/Head and Neck Surgery. Dr. LaBruna holds academic appointments as Associate Professor of Clinical Orolaryngology and Plastic Surgery at Weill Cornell Medical College and is an Attending Physician at The New York-Presbyterian Hospital. He also holds appointments at The Mount Sinai Hospital and Manhattan Eye, Ear and Throat Hospital. Dr. LaBruna is a Diplomate of the American Board of Plastic Surgery and the American Board of Otolaryngology.

Since 2001, Dr. LaBruna has been the Director of Facial Plastic Surgery in the Department of Otolaryngology at Weill Cornell Medical College. In this role, he trains medical students, residents and fellows in both departments of Otolaryngology and Plastic Surgery. He received an award for his outstanding teaching from the residents in Plastic Surgery in both 2004 and 2005. Dr. LaBruna has lectured both nationally and internationally on cosmetic surgery and facial reconstruction. He is also an Honorary Police and Fire Surgeon and has received honors from Commissioners Kelly and Scopetta. Dr. LaBruna serves on the Plastic Surgery National Board of Medical examiners which prepares questions for written examinations given to resident physicians.

Jaclyn A. Mucaria, M.P.A.

Ms. Mucaria is an experienced healthcare executive with a 20 year career in all aspects of hospital operations. She holds a Bachelor's Degree in Medical Technology from SUNY at Stony Brook, School of Allied Health Sciences and a Master's Degree in Public Administration from The Wagner School of Health Policy at New York University. She was an Associate Hospital Director at The Mount Sinai Hospital for twelve years where she directed areas such as diagnostic services, inpatient services, critical care, and outpatient services. Since 2000, she has been with New-York Presbyterian Hospital where she is the Vice-President for Ambulatory Care and Patient Centered Care. She is committed to serving the health needs of the community, especially the underserved population. She is also passionate about improving patient satisfaction and in her role as VP, leads an organizational effort to create a more patient and family centered culture.

We hope that you will enjoy reading this book as much as we enjoyed writing it.